WHOLEY COW

IT WORKS!

A Holistic Guide To Eating
And Recovery From Iron Deficiency

Barbara Rodgers

Wholey Cow It Works!

A Holistic Guide to Eating and Recovery from Iron Deficiency

The content of this book is for general instruction only. Each person's physical, emotional and spiritual condition is unique. The instruction in this book is not intended to replace or interrupt the reader's relationship with a physician or other professional. Please consult your doctor for matters pertaining to your specific health and diet.

To contact the author, visit
http://barbararodgersonline.com/

ISBN Number: 978-1-7327080-1-3

Printed in the United States of America
Cover Design: Sara Gamayunov

Interior Layout: Barbara Rodgers
barbararodgersonline.com

This book is dedicated to the billions of people who suffer with
iron deficiency and its many symptoms.
May you find comfort, peace and healing.

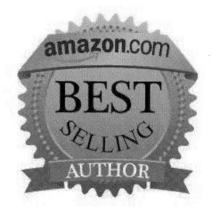

Acknowledgments

First of all I would like to thank God for guiding me on this journey and inspiring me to share what I learned to help others heal. Thank you for your divine goodness, ever present love and divine mercy.

I would like to thank my husband and daughters for your love and support. I am so grateful and very blessed to have you in my life.

I would also like to thank my daughter, Sara, for doing the photography for the cover of the book. I appreciate your creative skills.

Table of Contents

Introduction 9

Chapter 1: Lost The Pep In My Step 13

Chapter 2: Iron Deficiency 101 19

Chapter 3: Pump It UP—Treating Iron Deficiency 29

Chapter 4: Eating For Iron Deficiency 37

Chapter 5: What's Your Gut Got To Do With It? 63

Chapter 6: I Am Iron Man? Exercise and Iron Deficiency 77

Chapter 7: Dealing With The Symptoms 83

Glossary of Terms 105

Recipes 109

About The Author 137

Resources 139

Introduction

If you've picked up this book, you probably are suffering from iron deficiency, suspect you might be or know someone who has been diagnosed with it, but...

Who knew so many people out there aren't aware of the condition and what it involves, let alone how devastating some of the symptoms can be?

I was one of these people, until I was diagnosed with it myself a few years back and it hit me hard. I've always been a high-energy person and go-getter, so I was completely taken aback when I couldn't do some things I was used to doing, nor at the same pace. It actually affected me so much, that it led me on a path of learning more about nutrition and writing my first book, *Wholey Cow A Simple Guide To Eating and Living*. What I discovered was not only can eating the right foods help build iron levels, but can also help prevent and cure many illnesses and disease.

In my first book I touched a bit on my experience with iron deficiency and how it inspired me to become a Certified Integrative Health Coach and want to help others live healthier lives. After studying over 100 different dietary theories, I discovered many diets have commonalities and I used those commonalities to come up with 7 guiding principles for anyone to use to live a healthy lifestyle. After writing this book, however, I realized I wanted to write another book specifically geared for those suffering with iron deficiency so I could share more about my experience and approach to healing.

Overcoming iron deficiency takes time and definitely doesn't happen overnight! In fact, it can be quite a lengthy process for some individuals. Many people get discouraged, stressed out and don't necessarily know where to turn for support. Unfortunately, doctors aren't much help when it comes to the symptoms that go along with iron deficiency. Others don't grasp how many of the symptoms can wreak havoc on your body, as well as your emotions, especially when you might appear to look well. More education is definitely needed on the topic. Many doctors are well-informed about anemia, yet others don't realize iron deficiency itself can have many of the same markers. Low iron storage levels are often a red flag for symptoms, but this is sometimes overlooked by some physicians, especially when an individual's hemoglobin levels are in a set normal range.

After dealing with the ailment for a number of years and participating in various forums with others who suffer with iron deficiency, it became clear to me that a large number of people need help. I soon realized that some of the strategies that worked for me could help others too.

ARE YOU AWARE?

"Research suggests as many as 80 percent of people in the world don't have enough iron in their bodies. It also suggests that as many as 30 percent of people have anemia due to prolonged iron deficiency."[1]

Many people struggle with a multitude of symptoms, yet aren't given much guidance other than to take an iron supplement and eat more iron-rich foods. That is exactly what I was told and was sent on my way. Little did I know the road to recovery would be long and trying and completely change me!

Feeling extremely out of sorts with my symptoms, I was determined to get back to my normal self as soon as possible. I have always been very active, so I kept trying different things to keep me going and keep my spirits up. Many people don't understand the severity of symptoms iron deficiency can cause and the toll they can take on an individual. Like a lot of other people, I assumed taking an iron supplement would be a quick-fix and I would be feeling like myself in a few weeks. Boy was I wrong! I had no idea that brain fog, lethargy, irritability and more would plague me for longer than I cared. It was starting to wear on me, but I was determined to push through the symptoms that plagued me the most and kept looking for ways to make me feel like my own self.

For many people, it takes months and months to feel better. For others, it takes years and still others can't seem to shake it. Everyone wants a "magic pill" to feel better, but unfortunately it doesn't work that way with iron deficiency. Iron infusions may help some individuals and are prescribed in certain cases; however, they don't always produce lasting results and can cause side effects of their own. Most likely your body didn't become iron deficient overnight, so it makes sense that it needs an ample amount of time to replace what was lost. It's a process, so you need time to recuperate and feel balanced again. While dealing with many of the symptoms can be challenging, especially when your body is fatigued and you can't think straight, there are things you can do to feel more comfortable to get through it.

This book provides a holistic approach to healing from iron deficiency by focusing on a variety of natural healing modalities, including eating more whole foods and...

Wholey Cow It Works!

Each chapter is designed to inform you and guide you to recovery. From piecing together the symptoms, getting a diagnosis, conventional and alternative treatment options, choosing the right foods to build iron, practicing self-care techniques and more, this book will help lead you back to your whole, healthy self.

CHAPTER 1

Lost the Pep in My Step

"Energy and persistence conquer all things."
—Benjamin Franklin

Realizing Something Is Wrong

Most people live busy lives and often find themselves running from work to some other event. Whether it's a child's sporting event, a meeting, the gym or some other activity, people are frequently busier than they care to be. This was me a number of years ago. My husband and I owned a successful small business that took up a lot of time. While this kept me focused and engaged, I needed more to occupy my day, especially after my kids went off to college. I've always been an active person and love to exercise. I sometimes walked twice a day, went to the gym frequently, played tennis, practiced yoga and was involved in various other activities. I was one of those people that just had to keep moving.

I kept myself busy and thrived doing so until something inside of me changed. I first noticed a change in my energy early in 2013; although I am quite sure it dropped even earlier, but I brushed it off as overdoing it.

Like many other people, I wasn't paying attention to the signs my body was giving me. All of a sudden, I found myself getting fatigued rather easily, which was unusual and definitely something I wasn't used to. It didn't take long until my two walks a day turned to one. I just didn't seem to have the energy I used to and found myself skipping a walk in the evening. As time went by, my walks got shorter too. I found myself either turning around or going a shorter route. Additionally, I noticed I got extremely tired when cleaning my house. Cleaning never bothered me before, so I found this strange. In fact, cleaning used to give me energy. I've always been somewhat of a "neat freak" and habitually straightened things up. As my body became more run down, I noticed I started to get irritated when I had to clean, especially when there were a lot of people around. I suddenly found cleaning exhausting. Moreover, I started to become lax with my cleaning routine at home and no longer felt like the energizer bunny.

Being tired and experiencing fatigue is common place for those who suffer with iron deficiency. As a matter of fact, feeling worn out is one of the most common markers for the ailment. Unfortunately, a lot of individuals just dismiss it as stress or being part of life. Many people don't put two and two together until other symptoms develop.

> ### ARE YOU AWARE?
> *Being tired and experiencing fatigue is common place for those who suffer with iron deficiency and is a common marker for the ailment.*

More Symptoms

Although I didn't realize it at the time, I started to develop other symptoms too. I've always been a fairly optimistic person, but I started to become edgy and irritable. It didn't take long before my family picked up on the increased moodiness, anger and personality changes I was experiencing. I noticed it too, but I assumed it was hormonal and most likely related to perimenopause. I also began to worry more and felt an unease I never felt before in my life. Moreover, I started having trouble making decisions and began to lose my self-confidence and self-esteem. I was very timid and shy as a child and suddenly felt myself reverting back to this behavior. I felt overwhelmed, insecure and my health fading. This led me to become more withdrawn and feel alone.

Many people who suffer with iron deficiency have issues with anxiety. They may feel worried, agitated, irritable and may have trouble sleeping. That's because when iron is low, it can decrease oxygen availability and may cause disturbances in the brain creating a variety of symptoms. In fact, one study out of Japan found a connection between vitamin deficiencies and mental health and specifically linked low levels of iron and vitamin B6 to anxiety, panic attacks and hyperventilation. This makes sense, as both iron and vitamin B6 play an important role in how serotonin is synthesized. Serotonin is responsible for triggering pleasure centers in the brain and is known as the happy hormone. It is easy to see how one may not feel right if their iron, vitamin B6 or other nutrients are low or off.[2]

Besides that, I began to misplace things and just didn't seem to be able to think clearly. One day I caught myself throwing my hair brush in the garbage instead of putting it my vanity drawer. I also found myself throwing silverware in the garbage when unloading my dishwasher instead of the kitchen drawer where it belonged and putting dishes in the wrong cupboards. I know everyone can have a brain lapse from time to time, but I seemed to be having more and more of them. When I lost my eye glasses, I became alarmed. I wondered if I inadvertently threw them in the garbage like I had caught myself doing with other things. I just couldn't remember. Although I looked high and low for them, they never turned up. This was disturbing to me, as I rarely lost anything, let alone a pair of eye glasses. I also lost my wedding ring around the same time. I am pretty sure it fell in the tub while I was taking a bath and went down the drain, but I started to wonder about that too. I didn't know for sure and was having a hard time remembering. What's more, I recall going to work and staring at my computer. I couldn't seem to concentrate. It took me much longer to finish projects and writing became difficult for me, which was unusual and something I typically enjoyed. Ideas usually just came to me, but were few and far between. I also noticed I missed paying bills, which was something I always kept on top of. This really concerned me, so I started setting up reminders on my computer to try and prevent it from happening.

Many women who are iron deficient complain of poor concentration. That's not surprising as studies show that even moderate iron deficiency can impair a woman's thinking. In fact, in one study a group of women were shown an arrangement of pictures on a computer screen and then asked to recite what they saw in the grouping. On average, those with normal iron levels missed only a small percentage, while those with iron deficiencies missed twice as many as the normal iron level group.[3] Having an iron deficiency can disrupt brain functioning and may have an effect on the production of the brain chemicals dopamine and serotonin, which are often referred to as feel good hormones. Without enough iron in the brain, there are problems with neurotransmitter signaling, which can cause all sorts of cognitive and neurologic problems and symptoms.[4]

On top of everything else, I noticed my hair had been falling out over the last year or so and it really bugged me. No one really noticed because I have a lot of hair, but it felt different to me, especially on the sides of my head. I was very self-conscious and wanted it to stop. I was also worried it would continue to the point where it was noticeable by others.

Many people who have iron deficiency and iron deficiency anemia experience hair loss, which can be quite devastating for women. Some people notice more strands falling in the sink or shower. Others have noticeable thinning, bald spots or sections of hair falling out. Some individuals resort to wearing hair pieces or wigs to cover their thinning hair, which can be humbling for a woman and can promote self-consciousness. Many people who are affected with hair loss often wonder if their hair will start to grow back and, if so, ...when? The good news is with proper iron supplementation and eating an iron rich diet, hair does grow back in most cases for most individuals.

Hit Me like a Ton of Bricks

And then it hit me like a ton of bricks! I was so tired and fatigued that all I wanted to do was sleep. Even when I wanted to do other things, my body wanted rest, so I often found myself falling asleep on my coach. I knew something was wrong, and I was bound and determined to figure out what it was. Thankfully my intuition kicked in as I started thinking about all of the symptoms I was having—the tiredness, fatigue, poor concentration, memory issues, anxiety, heavy periods and hair loss. I began to wonder if all of these things could be related to the iron in my body. After doing a little online research and reading a bunch of articles, I was convinced I had a problem with the iron levels in my body and made a doctor's appointment to find out for sure. I wanted more than anything to find out what had happened to my old peppy self.

Wholey Cow Affirmations:

What I am feeling is temporary.
I give my body permission to heal and rest.

CHAPTER 2

Iron Deficiency 101

"Knowledge is power."
—Sir Francis Bacon

While everyone gets run down from time to time, being tired all of the time is not normal and could be a sign that something is wrong. Many people these days live fast-paced lives, eat the wrong types of food and are busy with work, family and other commitments, which can contribute to stress and fatigue.

If you are a person who suffers from constant sleepiness, irritability and gets fatigued easily, you may be iron deficient. You may also suffer from iron deficiency anemia, which is a condition in which your blood lacks adequate healthy red blood cells and is typically caused by an insufficient amount of iron in the body. The symptoms can be mild to severe and they usually develop over a period of time. Unfortunately, many people don't realize they have an iron deficiency and may attribute their troubles to something else such as stress, a hormonal imbalance, another malady or just daily living. It is estimated that 1.6 billion people globally suffer from iron deficiency. That's a lot of people and a lot of education to get out to those suffering with the condition, as well as the general public. Developing nations are especially at risk. In some areas, almost half of the population is affected. In the United States, it is a common problem for both women and children. In fact, 700,000 toddlers and 7.8 million women suffer with an iron deficiency in the U.S. alone. Pregnant women, the elderly and children are often at risk. Iron deficiency is a common problem for menstruating women, as well. In particular, women experiencing heavy periods during perimenopause are often affected by the condition. Additionally, it is a common problem for teenage girls who have poor dietary habits, which can lead to fatigue, extreme tiredness and more. A small percentage (2 %) of men are affected with iron deficiency anemia too.[5]

Role of Iron for a Healthy Body

Iron plays a big role in how your body functions and how you feel. Some key roles iron plays for health include: blood oxygenation, energy production, building muscles, skin and hair, maintaining a healthy immune system and proper brain functioning. Unfortunately, your body can't produce iron on its own. The only way we get iron is through the food that we eat and some drinking water that may contain minerals. That is why it is important to include plenty of iron-rich foods in your diet for optimal body functioning and to avoid iron deficiency. (See Chapter 4: Eating For Iron Deficiency.)

> ### ARE YOU AWARE?
> *"Iron is an essential mineral needed for blood production. Your body needs iron to produce hemoglobin, which in turn is needed to carry oxygen throughout your body and cells. Our main sources of iron come from plants and animals, although some processed foods are fortified with iron."[6]*

Iron to Oxygenate Your Blood
One of the most important roles that iron plays is to oxygenate your blood. Iron works with heme synthesis, which forms hemoglobin in your body. When you have healthy hemoglobin, oxygen is transported easily to the lungs, other body tissues and the brain so your body can properly

function.[7] Iron is also needed to keep your body warm. That is why many who suffer with iron deficiency complain of being cold all the time, or have cold hands and feet. I can attest to that, and it is no fun having cold hands and feet! Being cold all of the time and feeling like you can't warm up can be a miserable feeling.

Iron for Energy

Iron is critical for building muscles and keeping your energy levels up. Without enough iron in your body, you may feel tired or become fatigued easily. Many people may not realize what is causing their fatigue immediately, but chronic tiredness is usually a tell-tale sign of iron deficiency and more than likely other symptoms will develop. In order for your body to use energy, food has to be broken down. Iron plays a crucial role in this process by converting food to energy, and those without enough iron can become easily tired and fatigued. That is why it is important to have enough iron stores in your body.

Iron for Health and Well-Being

Iron helps your body maintain a healthy immune system. We are exposed to germs on a daily basis and having a healthy immune system helps protect against germs that may harm us and cause illness. Iron is needed for immune cell reproduction and maturation, which works to keep us healthy. If your body is low on iron, you might not be able to fight off infections as fast as others and your body may take longer to heal and recover from various illnesses, especially colds in the winter months.[8]

In addition, iron is needed for proper cognitive functioning. Memory, attention, problem solving and learning functions are all affected by low iron. Many people who are iron deficient or suffer with iron deficiency anemia often complain about poor concentration and may have trouble thinking clearly. Others may suffer with brain fog, especially in the morning. My brain fog often lifted in the afternoon, but some individuals experience brain fog throughout the day.

Diagnosing Iron Deficiency

If you are concerned you might have an iron deficiency, it is important to schedule a visit with your doctor. Your physician should ask you various questions about your health and symptoms. Most likely they will run a blood test to see if your hemoglobin level is low to determine if you have iron deficiency anemia. Hemoglobin will vary for men, women and children and there is a set normal range for each. "The problem is that most primary physicians screen for iron deficiency by testing for anemia. Unfortunately, these screening tests fail to identify people with mild to moderate iron deficiency, since iron stores will become almost completely depleted before your blood count drops."[9] Many people, however, exhibit symptoms way before this happens and may not be anemic albeit have the same symptoms.

If your hemoglobin levels are normal, yet your symptoms match many of those of iron deficiency anemia, make sure your doctor also tests your ferritin, which is a blood cell protein. A ferritin test will determine the amount of iron stored in your body. It is possible to have a normal hemoglobin level and still be iron deficient.

I am thankful that my gynecologist tested my ferritin levels. My iron stores were practically depleted, which left me feeling down, fatigued, cold, tired, suffering from hair loss and more. When tested, my ferritin level was at 2.5 nanograms per milliliter (ng/mL), which is quite low. The standard set range for ferritin is listed below.

Standard Ferritin Range

Normal Ferritin Range For Men:
20 to 500 nanograms per millimeter (standard unit)

Normal Ferritin Range For Women:
20 to 200 nanograms per milliliter (standard unit)[10]

It is sad that some people with iron deficiency go undiagnosed and are sometimes told by their doctor that their symptoms are all in their head. Doctors seem to be all over the board as far as diagnosing iron deficiency. It is disappointing that there is such a disparity on diagnosing parameters between various doctors. Functional medicine doctors and naturopaths often take a different approach and dig deeper. Their philosophy typically is to look for the root cause of a problem. Many of these practitioners have a different view point when it comes to the so-called "normal" readings. Many believe the standard ranges are way too low and look for an individual's ferritin level to climb well beyond the normal low set range of 20 ng/mL. Unfortunately, there can be variance among functional medicine doctors and naturopaths, as well. Let's take a look at an example below.

One functional medical doctor I came across explained her philosophy and broke iron deficiency into three stages, but the numbers were still on the low end of the spectrum.

First Stage: The first stage is usually mild and will show ferritin levels between 10 to 15 ng/mL. Individuals can exhibit various symptoms that some conventional doctors may dismiss or not necessarily recognize as a marker for iron deficiency.
Second Stage: The second stage occurs when an individual's ferritin drops below 10 ng/mL, in which a variety of symptoms can occur. Some functional medicine doctors flag anything under 30 ng/mL.
Third Stage: The last stage is when there is no longer any iron in the bone marrow and all stores are depleted. At this point, red blood cell production and hemoglobin typically drop, making a person obviously anemic. In this final stage, severe symptoms often show, leaving a person feeling exhausted.[11]

Although the idea of stages is a good framework, everyone is different and comes from various ethnic backgrounds. Many individuals exhibit symptoms at much higher ferritin ranges than just at the low end of the standard range spectrum. Some other naturopathic and functional medicine doctors believe individuals can exhibit symptoms of iron deficiency with ferritin levels less than 80 ng/mL and will prescribe iron supplementation or other treatment plans at this point.[12] I heard in several iron deficiency anemia forums that some hematologists believe ferritin numbers should be above 100 ng/mL, especially for women who still menstruate. This thinking is quite contradictory to most Western medicine doctors, yet would be beneficial to a lot of people who are suffering through symptoms and don't know why.

Notwithstanding, there are some clinical studies that back this up. In fact, one case study showed when determining iron deficiency, it is vital not to rely on results from just one test, but instead necessary to look at the entire picture for the individual (e.g., what symptoms is the patient exhibiting). Treatment should be observed and the individual should be re-tested over time, with the goal of reaching ferritin markers of >100ug/L. Treatment and testing should continue until any signs and indicators of the ailment subside.[13] Just think of the difference a holistic look could make in the lives and health of so many suffering from symptoms of iron deficiency if this became the norm.

Common Iron Tests

Some common tests used to determine iron levels in the body include the following:

Common Iron Tests

Hemacrit Test
A hematocrit test measures the percentage of red blood cells in the blood. It is part of a Complete Blood Count (CBC) test and is typically given to diagnosis both anemia and iron deficiency, as well as other vitamin deficiencies, dehydration and some other diseases.[14]

Serum iron Test
A serum iron test measures how much iron is in the serum or liquid of your blood, meaning what is left after both the red blood cells and clotting factors are removed from it.

Transferrin Test
A transferrin test will measure the direct amount of transferrin found in the blood. Transferrin is a blood cell protein that binds or fastens to iron so it can be transported throughout the body.

Iron-Binding Capacity
TIBC: (Total Iron Binding Capacity)
This test measures the total iron that can be bound to protein in the blood.

UIBC: (Unsaturated Iron Binding Capacity)
This test measures the reserves of transferrin, meaning what has not been saturated with iron.

Transferrin Saturation: This shows the percent of transferrin that is saturated with iron.

Serum Ferritin:
A serum ferritin test shows the amount of iron stores in the body.[15]

Causes of Iron Deficiency

Iron deficiency can result from numerous different causes, including lack of iron in your diet, iron absorption issues, or blood loss in the body from an ulcer, polyp, cancer or some other illness. It can also be caused by heavy periods in women, especially during perimenopause. Without enough iron, the body can't produce hemoglobin, which helps carry oxygen throughout the body and a multitude of symptoms can occur. [16]

Common Symptoms of Iron Deficiency and Iron Deficiency Anemia

Common symptoms of iron deficiency and iron deficiency anemia include:
Fatigue, disorientation, memory issues, moodiness, irritability, depression, hair loss, anxiety and sleepiness.

Other symptoms:
Headaches, heart palpitations, restless legs, chest pain and more.

Iron deficiency is the most common nutritional deficiency throughout the world and results from too little iron in the body. If you are suffering from one or more of these symptoms, see your doctor as these expressions can manifest as a number of maladies. Make sure you ask for a full gamut of iron testing, instead of just testing for anemia. If it is determined you have an iron deficiency, you can take steps to begin the road to recovery.

Wholey Cow Affirmations:

I am not alone.
My symptoms are my body's radar system to reach
for help and begin the healing process.

CHAPTER 3

Pump It UP—Treating Iron Deficiency

"Strength doesn't come from what you can do. It comes from overcoming the things you once thought you couldn't."
—Rikki Rogers

I am not sure if you are old enough to remember the old "Geritol" commercials that ran in the 70s, but I remember them vividly. They were popular when I was growing up and appeared on television frequently. I especially remember seeing the commercials while watching the Lawrence Welk Show, which aired on Sunday evenings. I believe Lawrence helped make them popular with his famous tag line he used when pausing for a commercial break...

"And now, a word from our sponsor, Geritol."

Frankly, as a kid, I didn't really know what Geritol was, but came to the conclusion that it was some sort of supplement for old, tired people. I do, however, remember it was advertised as, "with or without iron." These commercials ran for quite a number of years, and then all of sudden, seemed to disappear, just like the show. Nowadays, you don't hear much advertising on TV regarding iron and supplements, at least not the way Geritol was promoted in the 70s. In fact, I personally can't remember one commercial on television for a supplement promoting iron since those Geritol commercials ran all those years ago. It's kind of sad since iron deficiency affects such a large portion of the population. We definitely could use more awareness and education about the importance of iron in our diet. Thankfully I do see some promotion on some social media.

Everyone needs an ample amount of iron in their diet, whether they have an iron deficiency or not. Iron is needed in order for your body to function properly and optimally. While most people do get enough iron from the food they eat, many individuals do not. If you are concerned about not getting enough iron in your diet, you might want to consider taking a multi-vitamin with added iron to prevent an iron deficiency, especially if you are a woman.

> ### ARE YOU AWARE?
> *Everyone needs an ample amount of iron in their diet, whether they have an iron deficiency or not. Supplementing with a multi-vitamin with added iron may help prevent iron deficiency.*

Iron Supplements
If your doctor determines you have an iron deficiency, don't worry, it is treatable. Your doctor will most likely prescribe taking iron supplements, which should help pump up your iron levels and bring them back to a normal range so you can start feeling more like yourself again. Your doctor may recommend a certain dosage and particular brand, depending on your diagnosis, situation and testing levels.

Over-The-Counter Options
Most over-the-counter iron supplements contain around 25 mg of iron, although you may also be able to find some iron supplements with higher doses of iron. Iron supplements should be taken with food and a vitamin C supplement, or some sort of citrus food to help avoid stomach upset and aid in the absorption process. There are many brands and options of

iron available to choose from, so you may want to get some suggestions from your doctor to start.

Tablets/Capsules/Liquid

Iron comes in a variety of forms including: tablets, capsules, and liquid. You may have to try a few different options to find the form and brand that works best for you. Some iron supplements can cause bloating, nausea, stomach cramps and dark stools, which can be uncomfortable and hard to deal with at times. The best thing to do is to play around to find one that works best for you. I used a number of forms of iron and brands before finding a vegetable-based iron capsule that worked best for my body. It didn't seem to cause as much bloating or the constipating affects some of the other varieties I tried seem to have. I also liked that fact that it was made with whole foods. Keep in mind that everyone is different and your iron supplement of choice might be different from mine or someone else's choice.

Tablets and capsules are generally easy to take. If you have trouble swallowing pills, some capsules can be broken apart and taken with food. Try pouring the capsule in a smoothie, juice, yogurt or some other food such as oatmeal.

Liquids are easier to ingest and may be a better option for some individuals. Some people find that liquid iron is easier to absorb. I tried a liquid form for a while, but I didn't like the bloating it caused. Again, remember everyone is different, so you may have a different experience. Keep in mind that some liquids do not contain as much iron as some capsule forms, so you might have to take the liquid more often to increase the amount. Make sure you check with your doctor for proper dosing amounts, as this is based on your iron testing levels and diagnosis.

Prescriptions

If your iron levels are extremely low or you are anemic, your doctor may give you a prescription for a higher dose iron supplement. Prescription dosages typically vary, as they are based on the individual's various testing and circumstances. Make sure you follow your doctor's recommendations and contact them if you have any questions, problems or concerns.

Dosing

Most doctors recommend taking iron supplements daily for iron deficiency or anemia. Recent studies, however, suggest that supplementing every other day may help with iron absorption, but further investigation is needed.[17] I have always taken my iron supplements daily and was able to increase my iron stores this way. I have heard that some people have good luck dosing every other day. If you want to give every other day dosing a try, make sure you check with your doctor and listen to your body before making any changes. If you start to feel sluggish, fatigued or start to notice other symptoms after changing your dosing, it may be a good idea to go back to taking your iron supplement every day. Again, check with your doctor. Keep in mind that this may not work for everyone.

Iron Infusions

Although many people can restore their health with diet and iron supplements alone, some individuals may require other treatments. Thankfully I was able to raise my iron stores by taking iron supplements and eating an iron-rich diet. Depending on the cause and the severity of the deficiency, some individuals may require iron infusions to boost their iron levels more rapidly. Others may have trouble tolerating over the counter supplements or have problems absorbing iron through supplements, so an iron infusion may be recommended. Supplementation may be prescribed after monitoring the results of an infusion.

Diet Recommendations

Additionally, your doctor will most likely suggest eating an iron-rich diet. This is important as it takes time to bring your iron levels back to a normal range and even longer to bring them to an optimal level. Remember in most circumstances, iron doesn't get depleted overnight. Eating a healthy diet, including plenty of whole foods, will boost your body's ability to build iron and function properly. We will discuss more on eating for iron deficiency in Chapter 4: Eating for Iron Deficiency.

Treatment Parameters

When it comes to iron deficiency, most doctors will look at your ferritin levels and compare them with the standard set range. The problem is that this range is wide spread and is based upon the general population, many of whom may be unhealthy themselves. It doesn't necessarily look at what is optimal for an individual to feel well and is far from an ideal range.

While some doctors recognize this and may treat a patient earlier than waiting until ferritin numbers are in the standard low range, there definitely is inconsistency among doctors and what number to treat at. In my research, I found ideal ferritin numbers to be all over the board. For example, on the Mercola website, I found an article stating, "An ideal level of ferritin for adult men and non-menstruating women should be between 40 and 60 ng/mL and you do not want it to be below 20 ng/mL or above 80 ng/mL."[18]

I found another site of an Osteopathic Physician who stated that optimal ferritin levels should fall between 30-40 ng/mL.[19] Additionally, I found some naturopathic doctors and functional medical doctors that strive for an optimal range of 80 to 100 ng/mL.[20] I also heard some hematologists aim for even higher outcomes in an Iron Deficiency forum. This is quite a contrast, but clearly striving for higher ferritin numbers could have a huge impact on the elimination of symptoms for many individuals suffering from iron deficiency. Perhaps down the road the standard ferritin range may be raised to benefit more individuals to help alleviate their symptoms. In the meantime, make sure you do your homework. If you are not getting the results you want, or aren't being heard, you might want to find another doctor and get another opinion. Looking at the big picture for your health and working to achieve optimal hemoglobin, ferritin and iron numbers should be a paramount concern.

Other Ways to Add Iron

Besides taking supplements and eating foods rich in iron, there are a few other things you can try to help increase your iron intake. Keep in mind that these items are not necessarily substitutes for eating an iron-rich diet or a replacement for iron supplements and other treatment options, but rather can be used as an add-on or in conjunction with prescribed treatment parameters.

Desiccated Beef Liver Supplements

If you are looking for an additional boost of iron in your diet, you might want to try taking a desiccated beef liver supplement. This is something I used for a period of time when my iron stores were super low. It helped provide a little pick-me-up on those days I was feeling extremely fatigued. Keep in mind that the iron content is quite a bit lower than iron supplements. The recommended dosage of the brand I used was 4 capsules, which contained 3 mg of iron total.

Note: If you have questions or concerns about supplementing with beef liver, talk with your doctor, functional medicine doctor, naturopath, acupuncturist or other care provider.

Beef Spleen Supplements

Taking beef spleen supplements is another thing you might want to consider to help build your iron. Beef spleen supplements contain more heme iron than what is found in desiccated beef liver supplements. Beef spleen can also be used in conjunction with taking iron supplements. I did not use beef spleen supplements as a replacement, but rather as an add-on, as it does not have near the amount of iron as found in most iron supplements.

One capsule of beef spleen contains approximately 2 mg of iron and the recommended dosage is six capsules.[21]

Some functional medical doctors may recommend trying this approach or recommend using the beef spleen along with other recommended iron supplements.

Note: As with desiccated liver supplements, if you have questions or concerns about supplementing with beef spleen, talk with your doctor, functional medicine doctor, naturopath, acupuncturist or other care provider.

Cast Iron Pans
Cooking with cast iron pans and other cookware may offer another way to add iron into your diet. In fact, some research suggests that using cast iron pans may help increase the iron content of many foods. I know this may sound kind of hokey, but apparently there is some truth to it, as iron from the pan can flake off during the cooking process and be absorbed by certain foods. While there is no clear-cut known amount of iron absorbed when using cast iron pans, some foods may pick up 2-6 mg according to one source I found.[22] While I like my cast iron pans, they are kind of heavy and do require a bit of maintenance.

Lucky Iron Fish
The Lucky Iron Fish is a cooking tool that some people swear helps build iron. The fish can easily be added to any liquid-based cooking along with some sort of citrus juice (lime, lemon or orange) or vinegar. The Lucky Iron Fish can be used in broth, soup or other sauces. You can also boil water with the fish for drinking if you want an additional boost of iron in your day.

Patience Is a Virtue
Although iron deficiency can be stressful and a challenge to deal with at times, bear in mind it is treatable. It is important to be patient and allow your body time to recover. If you are diligent with your iron supplements or other treatment plan and follow an iron-rich diet, your body will naturally heal over time. (See Chapter 4: Eating for Iron Deficiency for more information on eating for iron deficiency.)

Wholey Cow Affirmations:

Everyone is different.
I listen to my body and choose what works best for me.

CHAPTER 4

Eating for Iron Deficiency

"I'm strong to the finish, 'cause I eats me Spinach."
—Popeye the Sailor Man

What the Heck Should I Eat Now?

If you've been told you are not getting enough iron in your diet, you are not alone. Many people these days lack iron in their diet. While there are a number of reasons this can happen (poor soil, eating too much processed food, gut problems), the good news is eating the right foods can help build your iron. While eating for iron deficiency may sound like a challenge for some people, it doesn't have to be. All it takes is a commitment, small adjustments and a positive attitude to get you on the path to healing and recovery. Most people already include some iron-rich foods in their diet like meat, vegetables, fruit and grains. Others may eat a variety of processed foods that contain iron such as bread, cereal or pasta. The key is to become more aware of what you are eating and make a conscious effort to include more foods rich in iron in your diet.

Processed Foods vs. Whole Foods

Unfortunately, there isn't one food that can cure iron deficiency. Eating an overall healthy diet is the best way to build iron. Many people these days often look for good tasting, easy to prepare food and often turn to processed foods because they are convenient. Although some processed foods contain iron and other nutrients your body needs, they do not contain the same amount of nutrients or the quality you get from eating whole foods. Moreover, many processed foods contain additives and preservatives that can have harmful effects on your body. Some of these added chemicals can also be harmful to your stomach and can lead to a variety of problems including leaky gut, gastritis, iron absorption issues and more. (See Chapter 5: What's your Gut Got To Do With It?)

When I was diagnosed with iron deficiency, my doctor handed me a list of foods that were considered high in iron and recommended that I eat more of them to help build my iron stores. For the most part, I ate healthy, but I definitely wasn't getting enough iron in my diet. I also discovered I needed to eat more in general to get the amount of iron needed to build my iron. The list I was given included a variety food, which contained both processed foods and whole foods. After giving it some thought, I chose to focus on eating more whole foods, especially vegetables, as this was what I lacked the most. While I ate vegetables, I definitely wasn't eating enough of them nor including them at every meal. Sadly, this is common for many individuals, especially if you eat a Western diet that is filled with processed food and fast food. The truth is, it's hard for anyone to get enough vegetables and nutrients in their diet eating this way.

When buying processed foods, make sure you look for products that are fortified or enriched with iron to help build iron.

Ways Nutrients Are Added To Processed Foods

Fortification:
The process of adding iron or other vitamins and minerals, protein or other ingredient to a product after processing to make it more healthful.

Enriched Foods:
Enriched foods have nutrients originally found in the product but lost during processing added back in as a means to keep some of the original nourishment.[23]

Some examples of fortification include adding iron to cereal, folic acid to bread, Omega 3 fatty acids to eggs or adding vitamin D and calcium to orange juice. Some examples of foods that are enriched are flour, white bread and pasta. Fortified and enriched foods are not a bad thing. They were introduced in the 1930s and intended to help boost the value of certain foods as a way to help prevent a variety of health ailments.[24]

Over the years, many food manufacturers latched on to the idea and began adding more nutrients to their products. Food manufacturers often use packaging claims to draw our eyes to one or two nutrients in a product, such as iron or calcium, as a means to make more sales. These advertising techniques are quite effective and help the manufacturer gain market share. Keep in mind that not all products that contain iron are marked as such, so it is best to take a closer look at the product before making your product selections.

Read the Food Labels

If you are not doing so already, the best way to decipher what you are buying is to start reading the food labels. Processed foods aren't always the healthiest choice, but many people buy them because they are convenient to make, eat and buy. Additionally, they are often less expensive than many whole foods. It is no wonder so many of us reach for them when out grocery shopping. We live in a society that is fast-paced, so it's common for many people to eat on the go and lean toward buying foods that are quick and easy to make. Think frozen pizza, cereal, macaroni and cheese, soup, crackers, chips and more.

While getting extra iron in your diet is important when you are iron deficient, eating added sugar, hydrogenated oils and other chemicals is not and can create ancillary problems. Often times these added ingredients can be appealing to your taste buds, but may leave you craving more. Furthermore, many processed foods contain additives and preservatives that give them a longer shelf life, but who knows what they are doing to our bodies? Sad to say, but they can wreak havoc on your insides. (See Chapter 5: What's Your Gut Got To Do With It?) Additionally, many processed foods lack other nutrients that your body needs, such as vitamin B, vitamin C, calcium and more. Another thing of concern is U.S. government regulations allow a margin of error of 20 percent on food labels, so they can be deceiving.[25] That's a big percentage and one that can be significant when you are looking to add iron in your diet. That is why it is always a good idea to get the majority of your nutrients from whole foods such as beans, greens, seeds and grains.

It is hard to get away from processed foods, as there are thousands of choices. Besides that, they seem to be everywhere—from grocery stores and gas stations, to big box stores, drug stores and more. The good news is that you can make smarter choices when selecting packaged foods. In addition to checking if a product contains iron, here are some things to look for when reading food labels.

If the list is long and involved, try to avoid the product. It is always best to shoot for 5 ingredients or less when purchasing packaged foods. If you can't pronounce an ingredient, it is best to steer clear of it. It is hard to identify what you are eating if you are not familiar with the ingredient. Get in the habit of asking questions up front before buying a product. This way you'll be more apt to make healthier choices, which will help lead you to healing and recovery.

Heme Iron vs. Non Heme Iron

Another thing to take into consideration when selecting foods that help build iron is the type of iron the food offers. There are basically two types of iron found in food: heme iron and non heme iron. Heme iron is found in meat from animals that contain hemoglobin, such as chicken, beef and fish. While not everyone eats meat, it is the best choice for iron consumption as it is more readily absorbed by the body. Non heme iron, on the other hand, is found in plants and while it isn't as easily absorbed as heme iron, is still a good option. In fact, most iron in our diet is derived from non heme iron. Your body needs non heme iron and is what vegetarians solely rely on. Some non heme iron sources include kale, apples, quinoa, almonds and sesame seeds. Most iron supplements, as well as processed foods, contain non heme iron.[26]

Types of Iron

Good Sources of Heme Iron
Beef, chicken, oysters, turkey, ham, liver, salmon, eggs, shrimp, chicken liver, lamb and pork loin

Good Sources of Non Heme Iron
Apricots, beans, bread, broccoli, cereal, kale, molasses, nuts, potatoes, raisins, rice, spinach and strawberries[27]

Eat More Produce

One of the most important things you can do to add more iron in your diet and stay healthy is to eat more fruit and vegetables. Fruit and vegetables contain vital nutrients your body needs to function properly and fight off disease. Vegetables are key as many have high iron content, especially greens and cruciferous vegetables. They also contain other vitamins, minerals and antioxidants you can't necessarily get from other foods or supplements. Many also contain fiber, which aids in the digestion process, helps get rid of waste and keeps your body healthy.

As I mentioned earlier, I chose to focus on eating more fruit and vegetables to help me get my energy up as fast as possible. Don't get me wrong, I still eat processed foods. I just try and limit them and look for healthier choices. It's hard to get away from processed food entirely, as they are so prevalent in our society.

While most people include some produce in their diet, the majority of people don't eat enough vegetables and often eat only a few varieties. On top of that, many individuals are confused regarding which type of produce to purchase and their value. Many varieties of produce have their own set of health benefits, so it is important to get a good mix. It's always a good habit to fill your plate with plenty of bright colored foods to reap their many nutritional benefits.

Organic vs. Conventional Produce

When shopping for produce, recognize that many fruits and vegetables, while good for you, contain pesticides. It is unfortunate, but much of the produce today is heavily sprayed and contaminated with chemicals, which can affect your overall well-being. Some fruit and vegetables have more pesticides sprayed on them than others. Over time, eating contaminated fruit and vegetables may affect your gut, which can lead to a host of problems including absorption issues. (See Chapter 5: What's Your Gut Got To Do With It?) This is why it is important to pay attention to what you are eating and learn how to protect yourself from these hidden and harmful chemicals.

Organic produce is always your best bet, since it is grown without pesticides and harsh chemicals. If you are on a budget or can't afford organic produce, don't worry. Conventional produce is still a better option than filling your grocery cart or shopping basket with junk food items such as chips, crackers, cookies or soda pop, as they are more likely to contribute to illness and affect your gut health.

If you purchase conventional produce, make sure you thoroughly clean your fruit and vegetables before consuming them to help remove some of the pesticides. (Please be aware that some pesticides and chemicals can penetrate through the skins and peels in some types of produce.) If you are interested in learning more about pesticides in produce, you may want to take a look at the website for the Environmental Working Group (EWG). www.ewg.org

The EWG provides a FREE downloadable guide that contains a list of the most heavily sprayed produce, which is known as the Dirty Dozen. They also provide another list called the Clean 15, which contains those fruits and vegetables that are considered "clean" and safe to buy. Unless you prefer to buy all organic produce, you should feel comfortable buying the conventional produce items on the list.[28]

Both lists are updated yearly, as the information can change. It's a good idea to check back from time to time for the most accurate information and current lists.

Choose Healthy Fat

When it comes to adding fat into your diet, many people are confused and rightly so. There's a lot of conflicting information out there in regards to fat and many people don't know what to believe. These days, you can find people who try and limit their fat intake and others who are trying to load up on it (think—Keto Diet or Atkins Diet). Still others are stuck on the low-fat craze idea from the 90s and stock up on plenty of low-fat foods. Eating a diet rich in nutrients, including iron and fat, is important for overall health. Limiting fat in your diet is not a good idea and can have serious side effects on your body. Restricting fat can disrupt hormones, impair digestion, weaken your bones and muscles, affect your kidneys and compromise your immune system. Our bodies need fat to operate properly and perform peak functions. Besides that, some studies done on rats suggest that including more fat in your diet can increase iron absorption of both heme and non heme iron intake.[29] More research regarding fat and iron absorption in humans is needed. One thing is clear, if you are not supplying your body with the fat it needs, your body can suffer in a variety of ways.

Many grocery stores carry an abundant supply of low-fat foods. It's really not surprising, as food manufacturers latched on to the low-fat notion when we were all told that fat is bad for you. In turn, food manufacturers developed hundreds of different food products with less fat than original versions as a way to increase their sales and make more money. With an abundant supply of low fat food products, it's no wonder so many of us started buying them and thinking they were a good choice.

Unfortunately, when fat is taken out of a food product or reduced, something else is added to the product to make it taste similar to the original version. Fat plays a big part in how a food tastes and is hard to replicate.

Oftentimes sugar or other sweeteners are added in the product to help improve the flavor. Chemicals and preservatives are also added, which can wreak havoc on the body and your gut when consumed on a regular basis. New studies also show that the original thinking that fat affects our cholesterol and causes heart disease were flawed. In fact, fat is not bad and eating the right types of fat can actually speed up your metabolism, help balance your hormones and help you think clearer.[30]

It's unfortunate we were told for decades that fat was a bad thing and many of us turned to a variety of products that are literally toxic. Our bodies need fat to function properly and perform peak functions. Instead of depriving your body of fat by eating low-fat food products, you should look more at the type of fat you are eating.

There are a variety of fats found in foods including saturated fat, mono-saturated fat, polyunsaturated fat and transfats. Monosaturated fats (MUFAS) are the good fats that help your body function optimally—think plant-based foods. Trans-fats, on the other hand, are not so good and are found in animals and animal products, such as milk. Other trans-fats are found in a variety of processed foods, such as potato chips, corn chips, crackers, condiments and more. These products typically contain hydroge-nated oil, which is man-made and created using an industrialized process that converts vegetable oil into a solid form. Consider staying away or lim-iting your intake of these products, as hydrogenated oil has been proven to have ill effects on your body.

When out grocery shopping, make sure you not only look for foods that contain iron, but also foods that contain good fats (MUFAS), as your body needs this type of fat to heal and recover.

Some Healthy Fat Foods Include:

- Avocados
- Nuts
- Seeds
- Nut or seed butter
- Olives
- Dark chocolate
- Coconut oil
- Olives
- Olive oil
- Flax seed

Other Healthy Fats

You can find other healthy fats in a variety of fish including salmon and tuna. You can also find healthy fats in eggs, tofu, edamame, full-fat yogurt, full-fat milk, a variety of hard cheeses (e.g., Parmesan cheese) and lean cuts of grass-fed beef and pork.

Beware of Sugar

Most people love sugar. It is sweet, delicious, enjoyable, and tempting! For many people it is hard to pass up a chocolate chip cookie, piece of cake or donuts at the office. After all, they often satisfy a sweet tooth and provide a sense of comfort, especially if you are feeling fatigued and run down. The problem is that sugar has addictive properties, and may lead to eating more. While sugar may provide a boost of energy at first, you'll likely experience an energy crash after an hour or so, leaving you feeling worse.

When out grocery shopping, make sure you read the food labels and avoid those foods with a high sugar content, added sugar or have sugar listed as one of the first ingredients. Sugar is found in just about everything these days, so be on guard when selecting processed foods. It is also important to pay attention to what you are drinking. Many drinks are loaded with sugar and can contribute to an unhealthy gut, cause weight gain and leave you feeling even more fatigued and tired. Some culprits include soda pop, coffee drinks, juice and energy drinks. A 12 oz. can of Coke alone contains 39 grams of sugar and some coffee drinks contain even more. It is a much better idea to look for products that boost your energy and not drain it.

Beware of Excitotoxins

Everyone loves good, tasty food, but some people have a hard time knowing when to stop eating. While it is often blamed on lack of self-control, some research suggests this behavior can be attributed to eating too much overly processed food on a daily basis. Many packaged foods contain substances called excitotoxins that literally excite your taste buds and make you crave more. If you are not familiar with excitotoxins, they are chemicals (typically amino acids) that over stimulate your brain and can cause neurons to die when there is an overabundance.[31]

Some common excitotoxins include MSG (monosodium glutamate) and aspartame. Both are found in hundreds of different processed food items that you can find while walking down the aisles in your local grocery store. MSG is a flavor enhancer and is used in hundreds of food items like canned soups, vegetables, sauces, seasonings and more. It is also frequently added in Chinese food and other ethnic foods to spice it up and give it some zing. It can also be found in a variety of restaurant food. Some people have immediate reactions to MSG, including headaches, upset stomach or nausea. Other people may develop issues later without realizing the issues may be attributed to MSG. Still others may think a little MSG won't hurt them. The problem is that a multitude of processed foods contain MSG and you may be ingesting way more than you think. Food manufacturers often hide MSG in their products by listing it as another name, so even if you look at packaging labels to stay clear of it, you still may be ingesting this harmful substance. Unfortunately, there are more than thirty different names for MSG, so beware.

Some other names for MSG include the following:

- Potassium Glutamate
- Soy Protein
- Natural Flavoring
- Yeast Extract
- Yeast Food
- Hydrolyzed Plant Protein
- Hydrolyzed Vegetable Protein
- Spices
- Nutritional Yeast
- Carrageenan
- Textured Protein
- Natural Flavoring
- Artificial Flavoring
- And more[32]

Aspartame is another popular excitotoxin used in many food products. Aspartame is derived from the amino acid aspartate and is used to sweeten diet soda pop, coffee, yogurt, candy, gum, tooth paste and more. Aspartame has been shown to cause serious neurological problems such as headaches, seizures and sleep issues and may change your gut bacteria and cause a host of problems. (See Chapter 5: What's Your Gut Got To Do With It?)

Some other excitotoxins include domoic acid (found in farm-raised fish), casein (found in cheese), cysteine and L-BOAA. These excitotoxins are used to improve the flavoring in a variety of foods that we consume. Besides exciting your taste buds and making you want to consume more of a particular food, excitotoxins can cause a variety of other symptoms. Some individuals may develop headaches, chest pain, insomnia, arthritis, skin irritations and depression. Excitotoxins can also cause stomach problems, including diarrhea and constipation, and may disrupt your gut flora balance, which may lead to nutrient deficiencies.

Excitotoxins have also been attributed to some other ailments and neuro-logical disorders by scientists and clinicians including the following: migraines, Parkinson's, Alzheimer's, ALS (Lou Gehrig's Disease), seizures and Huntington's Disease.

The best way to avoid the harmful symptoms associated with excitotoxins is to steer clear of them. It is also a good idea to pay attention to sea-soning packets, bouillon, salad dressings and personal care items such as toothpaste, lotions and facial cleansers. To avoid excitotoxins, your best bet is to eat a healthy diet rich in whole foods.

Consider also making your own seasonings for tacos, chili, spaghetti and more by using single spices to make your own mix. You can also avoid excitotoxins in salad dressings by making your own using items such as olive oil, fresh herbs, spices and lemon.

Beware of Foods That May Inhibit Iron Absorption

Although most individuals who have an iron deficiency are eager to learn which foods help build iron, it is also important to familiarize yourself with those foods that may inhibit iron absorption. Unfortunately, this can be a problem with some non heme iron foods, including vegetables and grains. Luckily there are some ways to enhance iron absorption in certain foods. In fact, just paying attention to how you pair your meals, as well as being mindful of certain substances, can make a big difference. Following are a few ways to enhance your iron absorption.

Mix and Match Heme and Non Heme Foods

Recall that we discussed earlier how heme iron found in meat such as beef, chicken and fish is more easily absorbed by the body. If you pair a steak with a non heme food such as a spinach salad or rice, the heme iron found in the steak will naturally help enhance the iron in the spinach and rice, especially if you add a little lemon in your dressing (see below Add Acidic and Vitamin C Rich Foods).

Add Acidic and Vitamin C Rich Foods

You already learned earlier that it is important to take your iron supplements with vitamin C, as it aids in the absorption process. The same holds true for non heme foods. To help absorb more iron from your meals, it is always best to pair non heme foods including whole grains, peas, beans, and lentils with fruit or vegetables that have acidic properties or contain vitamin C. For example, you could add tomatoes to a stir-fry or soup. You could also add lemon or lime juice to your rice or quinoa.

Add Natural Sugars

Many people like to sweeten their oatmeal with sugar. A better choice is to top it with fresh berries, bananas or apples. This way you will be enhancing both the flavor and iron absorption. You will also get a boost of other nutrients added to you meal. You can also try adding fresh fruit, honey or coconut to a bowl of quinoa or top your whole grain toast with peanut butter and a few banana slices. There are many ways to naturally sweeten and enhance your non heme foods, so be creative.

Pay Attention to Tannins and Polyphenols

Tannins are substances that are naturally found in plants, leaves, bark or fruit. They typically have a bitter, acidic taste, yet offer a distinct flavor. Tannins can be found in some tea and wine and may restrict iron absorption in some foods when consumed together. Some other caffeinated beverages may block iron.

Polyphenols are chemicals found in plants that give them their coloring. They can be found in wine, chocolate, berries and some nuts. If you are concerned about iron absorption or are having issues, it is probably best to wait an hour or two after having your meal to enjoy a cup of tea or glass of wine. I honestly didn't worry about this too much and just enjoyed my cup of tea or glass of wine most of the time. I would do what feels best for your body.

Keep in mind that it is highly unlikely that the tannins themselves are a cause of iron deficiency, so it isn't necessary to avoid them altogether.

Pay Attention to Fiber, Phytates and Oxalates
Another thing you should pay attention to is phytates and oxalates found in a variety of fiber-rich grains and vegetables, as well as nuts. They can decrease the absorption of some non heme foods. Phytates typically are found in grains, legumes, nuts and seeds. Although many of these foods are rich in iron that benefits your body, the phytic acid found in them may cause absorption problems. To get around this, it is best to pair them with foods rich in vitamin C including tomatoes, limes and bell peppers. You can also remove some of the phytates from grains, beans and nuts by soaking them before cooking.

Oxalates are a natural occurring substance found in vegetables, fruit, nuts, seeds, grain, tea and more. In general, they are not bad and help support your metabolism. Some foods high in oxalates can cause issues with absorption and may accumulate in the body. Foods high in oxalates include spinach, kale, dark chocolate, beets and rhubarb. Many of these foods are also rich in iron, so you probably don't want to avoid them altogether. Like phytates, oxalates can be paired with other foods rich in vitamin C. You can also boil vegetables that are high in oxalates to remove some of the oxalic acid. Just make sure you discard the water. You can also eat foods rich in oxalates apart from your meal, so go ahead and enjoy your piece of dark chocolate or cup of tea a bit later and savor the flavor.

Separate Foods Rich in Calcium
Foods containing high amounts of calcium such as milk, cheese or yogurt can also affect the absorption of some non heme type foods. If you enjoy dairy, instead of avoiding it altogether, try eating dairy foods an hour or so later than your non heme meal to avoid any problems. Some other calcium rich foods that may be of concern include sardines, broccoli, almonds and rhubarb. Keep in mind that you can also pair them with acidic or vitamin C rich foods.

51

Separate Your Supplements

Multi-vitamins and other vitamins may also affect how you absorb iron. The reason being is that zinc, calcium and other vitamins may compete for the same binding site as iron. To avoid this potential problem, try taking your other supplements several hours after your iron. I try to take my iron supplements first thing in the morning along with a vitamin C supplement, and my other supplements an hour or two after breakfast.

Low Stomach Acid

Many people today have stomach problems and often turn to antacids and other medications to relieve acid reflux and other gut ailments. Many people who take antacids actually have low stomach acid instead of high stomach acid, which can negatively affect iron absorption and absorption of other vitamins. Taking excessive amounts of antacids or using them for long periods of time can also affect iron absorption. Moreover, elderly individuals tend to produce less stomach acid. If you fall into one of these categories, you may find that taking a hydrochloric acid supplement is beneficial.[33] (See Chapter 5: What's Your Gut Got To Do With It?)

> ## ARE YOU AWARE?
> *Many people who take antacids actually have low stomach acid instead of high stomach acid, which can negatively affect iron absorption and absorption of other vitamins.*

Note: If you have questions or concerns about supplementing with hydrochloric acid, talk with your doctor, functional medicine doctor, naturopath or other care provider.

Watch the Restaurant Food

Many people today eat out several times a week or more. While eating out may be fun and convenient, most restaurants serve large portions and often use ingredients that may not be the healthiest for your body. Unhealthy oils, high carbohydrate foods and sugar, are unfortunately often found in the majority of restaurant meals. A healthier option than going out to eat is to make more home-cooked meals. When you eat at home, you are in charge of what you serve and how it is prepared. You also have the opportunity to choose healthier ingredients, prepare foods you know are iron-rich and pair them with other foods that help aid absorption. You can also add other foods to your meal that are nutrient dense to help heal your body and lead you to recovery.

Keep a Food Journal

The best way to get to know how the foods you are eating affect you and if they are helping in your recovery process is to track what you are eating. Writing down what you eat not only is a great way to get to know yourself, but can also help you identify which foods give you energy and which foods don't. Keeping a food journal can also help uncover specific habits, patterns and cravings, as well as emotional triggers you might have with food. In addition, recording what you eat can help uncover foods that may leave you feeling fatigued, bloated or irritable. Journaling can promote healing by helping guide you to make better food choices.

Moreover, the information you record may help you uncover food sensitivities and foods that may cause gut irritation. Use the information you record as a guide to aid in the healing process. For instance, let's say you like to eat cereal for breakfast most days, but have a breakfast sandwich or oatmeal a day or two during the week. A lot of cereals are fortified with iron, so you may think that cereal is a good choice to help increase your iron. The problem is that many of us don't necessarily pay attention to the sugar content and long list of ingredients found in many cereals, which may have adverse effects on your body when consumed on a regular basis. When you record what you are eating and how it makes you feel, you may discover your favorite cereal may not be the best choice for healing. The breakfast sandwich and oatmeal also contain iron, as well as protein and other nutrients that should give you a boost of energy and sustain you longer. Adding fruit, nuts or coconut to your oatmeal will also provide other nutrients your body needs for healing.

Food Journal Example					
Date	*Time*	*Food Eaten*	*Meal/ Snack*	*Emotion Felt*	*Hunger Rating 1-5*
07/01/19	7:00	cereal, banana	break-fast	anxious/ hurried	3
07/01/19	10:30	candy bar	snack	sluggish	4
07/01/19	1:00	chicken sandwich, fries, soda pop	lunch	tired	5
07/01/19	3:00	carrots and hummus	snack	calm	2
07/01/19	6:00	steak, po-tato, bread, beans	dinner	relaxed	4
07/01/19	8:30	ice cream	snack	stressed	2
07/02/19	7:00	oatmeal	breakfast	calm	4

There are many options when it comes to food journals. You can create your own using a spreadsheet or table or just use a notebook and hand-write your entries. You can also download an app on your phone or find a template on Pinterest or Google. There are many options and no one right method. The most important thing is to pay attention to your body and become aware of which foods are helping you feel better and building your iron.

Iron-Rich Snacks

It is important to fuel your body with plenty of iron-rich food through-out the day if you are iron deficient. Obviously you want your meals to contain a good deal of iron and may want to consider including both heme and non heme iron sources, although it's not imperative to include heme iron. Besides that, it is important to incorporate several iron-rich snacks into your daily routine to help build iron in your body. While some individuals may struggle with what to snack on, there are a lot of healthy options. Some of the best sources of iron-rich snacks come from whole foods, including vegetables, as they contain vitamins, minerals and antioxidants your body needs to heal and flourish. Sweet vegetables in particular are a good choice, as they not only add a crunchy taste, but may help satisfy cravings for other sweets like cookies, cake or candy. Try adding carrots, bell peppers or snap peas as part of a healthy morning or afternoon snack.

Following are a few other good sources of iron-rich snacks you might want to try to include as part of your healthy fare.

Apricots

The apricot is considered one of the healthiest fruits in the world.[34] It is loaded with healthful nutrients and has many benefits. Apricots contain vitamin C, vitamin A, potassium and plenty of fiber. They also contain a healthy dose of iron, which is a vital element for muscle and brain health and also works to regulate body temperature. Although I like apricots, it wasn't a fruit I bought a lot of. When I developed iron deficiency, however-er, I began buying dried apricots to snack on. They are sweet and make a good, healthy snack.

Blueberries

Blueberries are a popular fruit and an important food to include in your diet if you suffer with iron deficiency. Blueberries not only taste good, but are loaded with phytochemicals, antioxidants and minerals. They also contain a healthy dose of vitamin C, which aids in iron absorption, as well as helps build immunity and fight inflammation. Blueberries also contain iron, which helps provide energy for your body. Blueberries contain other vitamins such as vitamin K, vitamin B6, potassium, magnesium, zinc and fiber, which help keep your body functioning optimally. Blueberries are a tasty treat and make a healthy snack anytime of the day.

Dark Chocolate

If you are a chocolate lover, you will love the fact that dark chocolate is rich in iron. Chocolate is sweet and satisfying and it's no wonder many people crave it. Chocolate is loaded with antioxidants that are good for your body. Chocolate is also rich in fiber and a number of other minerals including magnesium, copper, potassium, zinc and selenium, which can help give your body a boost of energy. Despite all of its health benefits, it is important not to over indulge. Stick to a square or two of good quality dark chocolate, as it does contain sugar and caffeine. Chocolate is also acidic, so large quantities aren't necessarily good for your gut. Keep in mind that milk chocolate and white chocolate do not have the same benefits as dark chocolate and have much more sugar, as well as food additives that may have adverse effects on the body.

Dates

Dates are loaded with a variety of antioxidants and nutrients your body needs. Dates are popular around the world, most often consumed dried and have been around since biblical times. Some nutrients found in dates include potassium, calcium, magnesium, phosphorous, vitamin B6, niacin and fiber. They are also a descent source of iron, which is needed for overall well-being.

Dates are sweeter than many other types of fruit you might be used to eating and contain plenty of natural sugars. Some natural sugars found in dates include glucose, fructose and sucrose, which your body easily processes into energy. Dates are convenient to eat and make a good snack to munch on after a workout or walk. They also work great for an afternoon pick me up or a boost of energy to get your day going. Instead of reaching for that power bar, try eating 2 to 3 dates.

Figs

When it comes to iron-rich snacks, figs are a power-house and definitely one that you may want to include in your diet. Although figs aren't as popular as some other types of fruit, they have been around since ancient times and are mentioned throughout the bible. Figs are a sweet treat and loaded with antioxidants, vitamins and minerals. Some nutrients found in figs include vitamin A, vitamin K, B vitamins and magnesium. They are also a good source of both iron and vitamin C, which is a good combination when you are looking to build iron in your body. Figs are also rich in fiber, which aids in the digestion process. Another bonus of eating figs is they help promote hair growth, since they are rich in zinc and copper, which help prevent hair loss. Try adding a few dried figs as a morning or afternoon snack to reap their health benefits.

Hummus

If you're looking for a rich, filling snack that's not so sweet, you might want to try hummus. If you're not familiar with hummus, it is a creamy, thick spread made from chick peas. Hummus is a popular Middle-Eastern food that has been around since ancient times. In some cultures, hummus is consumed with every meal. In the Western world, hummus is often enjoyed as a snack or served as an appetizer. Hummus has a host of beneficial nutrients that have medicinal affects for your body. Chickpeas have an array of vitamins and minerals including protein, copper and folate. They are also rich in iron and B vitamins. Additionally they are a good source of fiber, which aids in digestion. Hummus also contains tahini, which is made from ground sesame seeds and has nutritional benefits of its own. What's more, tahini is a good source of iron and beneficial to those with iron deficiency. For an afternoon pick me up, try eating some hummus with vegetables, crackers or pita bread.

Nuts
Nuts are a great snack food and are not only delicious, but nutritious. It is no wonder they are a popular snack choice for many people. Nuts are loaded with many healthful nutrients including protein, vitamin E, magnesium, selenium and copper. They also contain healthy fats (MUFAS) that your body needs to function properly. Many nuts are also rich in iron, which helps deliver oxygen to your cells. Try grabbing a handful of nuts to snack on to help build iron and boost your energy. Almonds, cashews, walnuts and hazel nuts are all good options.

Pumpkin Seeds
If you are looking for a crunchy, tasty snack to give you an added boost in the morning or afternoon, why not try some pumpkin seeds? Pumpkins are good for you and packed with a bunch of feel-good nutrients. Pumpkin seeds are a good source of iron and can help boost your energy. In addition, pumpkin seeds contain a variety of other nutrients including magnesium, zinc and copper, which some individuals who are iron deficient may also be lacking. Moreover, pumpkin seeds are high in fiber, omega 3 fats and protein. You can eat pumpkin seeds alone or add them to yogurt, smoothies and more.

Strawberries
Strawberries are a sweet, tasty fruit that many people enjoy. Strawberries are juicy, have a delightful flavor and are good for you. Strawberries are loaded with antioxidants that have inflammatory properties, so they are beneficial for arthritis, cancer, neurological disorders and other diseases. They also contain a variety of nutrients that are beneficial for your body and are considered a super food. Some nutrients found in strawberries include vitamin C, potassium, magnesium, protein, vitamin K and folate. Strawberries are a good source of fiber, which aids in the digestion pro-

cess. While strawberries don't contain as much iron as some other types of fruit, they do help contribute to iron absorption. This is due to the fact that strawberries contain a high amount of vitamin C (roughly 100 mg) and foods rich in vitamin C help individuals absorb iron. Snack on this tasty fruit and enjoy its many health benefits.

Eat With the Seasons

While you may have heard that eating seasonally is good for you, it is not some new idea or trendy movement. People have been eating with the seasons for centuries. Before global transportation and big business, people ate what was prevalent from the land. It was common place to eat what was harvested and available from the fields. Many root vegetables and grains were stored to eat during the winter months. People naturally enjoy produce such as tomatoes, cucumbers and watermelon during the summer months, or carrots, squash or pumpkin in the fall when they are abundant. While they naturally taste better, there are other benefits from eating seasonally.

Everyone likes fresh food. It not only tastes better, but has more nutritional value than when purchased and consumed out of season. That's because seasonal food doesn't need to be transported far. Oftentimes when produce is shipped, it is picked early and still needs to ripen. Chemicals may be used to enhance the ripening process and to assure the produce can be kept for a longer periods of time. Fresh produce, on the other hand, doesn't necessarily have all those chemicals and is much better for your body.

Eating seasonal food can save you money too. When produce is in season, there's a generous supply, so the prices tend to go down. Many farmers also supply local grocery stores with their harvest. Farmers markets are popular these days and provide another way to enjoy fresh produce. Additionally, having a garden and growing your own food is great way to include more fruit and vegetables in your diet during the growing season. That is, if you have the time and energy to maintain it, which may be tough if you are struggling with iron deficiency. Gardening certainly is something you can strive for down the road if it something that interests you.

They say "variety is the spice of life." Many people get stuck in a rut when it comes to eating and often eat the same things over and over. This can especially be true for some individuals trying to eat for iron deficiency. It is important to mix things up. Choosing seasonal foods not only will give your taste buds variety, but your body will benefit from a variety of different nutrients.

Seasonal foods provide vitamins and minerals your body needs for a particular season. For example, in the winter, citrus foods are plentiful and are high in vitamin C, which can help prevent colds and flu that you might be prone to if your body is run down. Citrus foods are also good to pair with some non heme iron foods as we discussed earlier. Winter vegetables such as potatoes and onions work well for comfort and warming foods, such as soups, stews and casseroles and are great to eat when you are feeling cold and can't seem to warm up.

Summer foods such as watermelon and cucumbers are considered cooling foods and help keep your body hydrated when it is hot. Lettuce, kale and peppers contain nutrients that provide energy and help keep you going.

Seasonal eating also gives you the opportunity to cook more. Remember—when you take the time to make your own meals, you're in control of what you buy and eat. Make sure you choose plenty of seasonal foods to add variety and reap their nutritional benefits for healing.

Wholey Cow Affirmations:

I am what I eat.
I choose foods that give me energy and provide
life-giving nutrients.

CHAPTER 5

What's Your Gut Got To Do With It?

"All disease starts in the gut."
—Hippocrates

If you are suffering with iron deficiency, by now you probably know that increasing your iron with supplements and food is important. Unfortunately, for some individuals, this is only part of the path to recovery. Many people who are iron deficient never find out the true cause of their problem. In some cases, where there is blood loss from an illness, polyp, ulcer or heavy periods, it is more obvious, but there still could be other underlying causes. Others may not be getting enough iron in their diet if they follow a strict vegetarian diet or eat the Standard American Diet (SAD), which consists mainly of processed and fast foods. If you don't fall into one of these categories you may be told you have iron absorption issues. But why is that and what causes it?

Getting to the Root Cause
That's a good question and one that isn't always addressed. Some people are diagnosed with gastrointestinal issues (GI), such as irritable bowel syndrome or inflammatory bowel disease that may affect how they

absorb iron and other nutrients. Others may have issues with their gut yet not be aware of it. This is a common problem these days and fortunately we are starting to hear more about how our gut health can contribute to our overall health.

Not everyone may realize, but there are trillions of bacteria located in your gut. The good news is that not all of the bacteria are bad. When most of us think of bacteria, we think of the bad bugs that make us sick. Your gut, however, houses both good and bad organisms that contribute to your overall health. Your gut plays a big part in your immune functioning, as well. In fact, it contains "70 percent of the cells that make up your immune system."[35]

Researchers have found that your gut and brain work together and there's a strong communication link. "Our brain and gut are connected by an extensive network of neurons and a highway of chemicals and hormones that constantly provide feedback about how hungry we are, whether or not we're experiencing stress, or if we've ingested a disease-causing microbe."[36]

> **ARE YOU AWARE?**
>
> *Your gut plays a big part in your immune functioning. It contains "70 percent of the cells that make up your immune system."[35]*

Your gut also passes messages back to your brain, which can influence your choices with food, mood and even behaviors. This is why it is important to have a healthy balanced gut. People with diverse microbiomes are more likely to feel healthy and vibrant, which is why it is important to keep your gut in good shape.

So What's a Microbiome?

A microbiome is "a community of microorganisms including bacteria, fungi, and viruses that inhabit a particular environment, such as in the gut or other area of the human body."[37] A microbiome is like a garden. A healthy garden contains nutrient-dense plants that are good for your body and flourish with water, sunshine and lots of tender loving care.

Without routine maintenance and TLC, weeds can spring up and can take over. When there are too many weeds, they can choke off the healthy plants, leaving them diseased or unhealthy. That's what happens in your gut when unhealthy bacteria and organisms take over, and it can lead to dysbiosis and inflammation.

What's Dysbiosis?

Dysbiosis is an imbalance in the bacteria of the gut, which can cause a variety of health problems and disease.[38] It can also lead to leaky gut, which happens when the epithelial cells of the intestinal wall break down and cause openings. These openings let food into the bloodstream where they are considered invaders and thus trigger an antibody reaction and inflammation. It also causes malabsorption of nutrients, such as iron, magnesium and others, and can lead to illnesses such as iron deficiency, anemia, Crohn's disease, food sensitivities, allergies, arthritis, lupus and other autoimmune diseases.[39]

Food Sensitivities

Food sensitivities seem to be prevalent these days and it's no wonder, as many people are eating the wrong types of food that can cause inflammation. Most people aren't aware they could have a food sensitivity and may attribute their issues to something else. If you are having gut problems you might want to explore food sensitivities, as they can cause inflammation, acid reflux and more. They can also contribute to absorption issues with iron and other nutrients. Many symptoms can be minor, but can contribute to fatigue, tiredness, brain fog, stomach issues and more. If you are concerned you might have some food sensitivities, you may want to consider doing an elimination diet to find out what foods may be causing your problems. Another option is to get some food sensitivity testing. Talk with your doctor, functional medicine doctor, naturopath or other practitioner for more information. Some common symptoms of food sensitivities include gas, bloating, acid reflux, burping, heartburn, GERD, brain fog, joint pain, unexplained rash, fatigue and more.

Multiple Vitamin Deficiencies

Some people who have iron deficiency may find they also are deficient in other vitamins. This makes sense as inflammation and dysbiosis can affect absorption of a variety of nutrients in your gut. Some people who have iron deficiency are also deficient in vitamin B12, folate, copper or vitamin D. If you suspect you have other vitamin deficiencies, make sure you check with your doctor for testing, as they may cause other problems. Since it is fairly common for people who suffer with iron deficiency to also be deficient in vitamin B12, I want to provide more information on that deficiency.

Vitamin B12 Deficiency

Vitamin B12 deficiency and iron deficiency have some common symptoms. Unfortunately, some people may suffer with both ailments and may not realize it. Some common symptoms of vitamin B12 deficiency include fatigue, brain fog, anxiety, depression, numbness and tingling sensations, especially in their hands or feet. Other symptoms such as cognitive impairment, personality changes, mental confusion and forgetfulness can also appear over time if left untreated.

Like iron deficiency, vitamin B12 deficiency can be caused from not getting enough of it in the diet. Some foods that contain vitamin B12 include meat, eggs, milk and other dairy products. Some processed foods such as cereal and bread are often fortified with vitamin B12. While most people get enough vitamin B12 in their diet, some people at risk include those who are malnourished, vegetarians, vegans and pregnant women who consume little or no animal products.[40]

Vitamin B12 deficiency can also be caused from poor absorption. As with iron deficiency, a vitamin B12 deficiency can be caused from stomach problems stemming from inflammation and low stomach acid. Ironically, vitamin B12 is needed to break down foods in the stomach and helps promote healthy bacteria in the gut, so it ends up being a double-edged sword for some individuals. Vitamin B12 is also needed for red blood cell formation, healthy metabolism, heart health, nervous system function and more.[41]

Vitamin B12 deficiency may also lead to vitamin B12 deficiency anemia, which can happen over time if the small intestine isn't absorbing vitamin B12 properly. Anemia of this type can be caused from a number of different things including celiac disease, Crohn's disease, stomach surgery, over growth of unhealthy bacteria in the stomach and a tapeworm. Still, the most common cause of vitamin B12 deficiency occurs when the body fails to produce a protein called intrinsic factor. This protein is very important, as it adheres to vitamin B12 and helps guide it through the small intestine and then on to the blood stream where it is absorbed and used. If you lack intrinsic factor, an autoimmune disease is most likely to blame. It can also be caused from an inherited condition that is passed down in families. Sadly without enough intrinsic factor your immune system will inadvertently strike against the cells in your stomach that produce it, creating all kinds of problems. This type of B12 deficiency is called pernicious anemia.[42]

Additionally, vitamin B12 deficiency can be caused from methylation issues. Vitamin B12 has a number of forms—cyanocobalamin and methylcobalamin being the most common forms. In order for our bodies to use it, the cyanocobalamin must be converted to methylcobalamin. Regrettably, some people have a problem converting it. On top of that, at least half of the population has a MTHFR gene mutation that makes them less able to methylate vitamin B12. Make sure you check with your doctor or functional medicine doctor for more information or testing if you suspect methylation problems with vitamin B12.[43]

If you suspect you have a B12 deficiency, make sure you get tested. The best way to test for a vitamin B12 deficiency is to have a methylmalonic acid test. If you suspect you have an inherited B12 condition, you will need further testing including testing for intrinsic factor.

What Causes Leaky Gut?

The world we live in today is much different than it was 50 years ago, so it it's not surprising both food and our environment can contribute to leaky gut. Other factors such as processed foods, factory farming and big business all play a role in how our society has changed and the foods we eat. While we have many more choices and technological advances, we need to take a hard look at how they affect our overall well-being and health.

Leaky Gut Contributors

There are a variety of things that can affect your gut microbiome and create an imbalance in the bacteria that causes leaky gut. Some common irritants include:

Eating a Western Diet

A Western diet (SAD) typically contains lots of processed foods and fast food. These types of food tend to be heavy on carbs and incorporate sugar-laden foods and unhealthy oils (e.g., transfats, hydrogenated oils), all of which can affect the bacteria in your gut and cause aggravation. Inflammation in the stomach can cause gastritis and other problems, all of which can lead to absorption issues and more.

Using a Lot Of Antibiotics or NSAIDS

Antibiotics can be hard on the stomach, as they kill both bad and good bacteria and can disrupt the balance of your microbiome. If you are person who has used antibiotics frequently and have low iron, you may want to look into healing your gut and adding more healing foods to your diet. (See Chapter 4: Eating for Iron Deficiency.) Over use of NSAIDS can cause stomach bleeding and ulcers, leading to leaky gut.

Birth Control

Birth control pills are popular for preventing pregnancy and other symptoms, such as painful periods, endometriosis and acne. Birth control pills, however, do have drawbacks. Like antibiotics, birth control pills can alter your gut microbiome and can create imbalance. If you use birth control pills or have used them recently, make sure you eat plenty of anti-inflammatory foods to help nourish and heal your gut. It is also a good idea to take a probiotic supplement to help promote healthy gut flora.

Taking Drugs That Lower Stomach Acid

Some medications can alter the flora in your gut and create an imbalance. Antacids, proton pump inhibitors and other medications used to treat heart burn and acid reflux can all contribute to leaky gut. Additionally, having acid reflux and heartburn itself can be sign that there is a bigger problem going on. Many people who take antacids actually have low stomach acid, not an excess of it. Additionally, it is fairly common to produce lower stomach acid with age. Individuals with low stomach acid may find taking a hydrochloric acid supplement more beneficial than taking antacids and other drugs. Hydrochloric acid helps break down food in the stomach and helps your body absorb nutrients. If you don't have enough stomach acid, you may not be able to absorb iron, vitamin B12 or other nutrients. If you work on healing your gut, however, absorption issues can be eliminated.

Alcohol

Alcohol is another culprit that can affect your microbiome. While it may be fun to have a few drinks now and again, overuse of alcohol, especially over time, can contribute to various diseases and a decline in health. To help avoid leaky gut and other issues, try cutting back on alcohol consumption or eliminate it all together.

Artificial Sweeteners

Artificial sweeteners are popular and are used to sweeten thousands of food products and beverages. Unfortunately, artificial sweeteners are loaded with chemicals your body doesn't necessarily know how to process. In addition, no one knows for sure what the long term effects of consuming artificial sweeteners are. Artificial sweeteners are also a common irritant for your gut and can wreak havoc on your microbiome. If you want to have a healthy gut, help eliminate absorption issues and restore gut balance, it is a good idea to steer clear of any artificial sweeteners such as aspartame, saccharin and sucralose found in a variety of processed foods, soda pop and other beverages. (See Chapter 4: Eating for Iron Deficiency.)

Gluten

Gluten is a protein made up of several peptides and can be found in a variety of grains including wheat, rye, barley and spelt. It is what gives bread and other baked goods its airy, light texture and dough that sticky feeling and consistency. Gluten can be found in many processed foods, as it works like glue and is often used as a thickening agent. These days we hear a lot about people having gluten sensitivity or developing celiac. That's because our food has significantly changed over the last 50 years or so. Whole grains have been a central part of the human diet since early civilization. Today's grains, however, are much different than grains of the past. Many grains today are genetically modified and treated with chemicals to help preserve them and give them a longer shelf life. It is no wonder that many people have developed food allergies, sensitivities and problems tolerating gluten as a result of the modifications. What's more, the gluten found in the majority of food we eat today can contribute to irritation of the stomach. In fact, antibodies that strike against unidentified and harmful substances in the stomach are often formed in those who have gluten sensitivities. This creates permeability and nutrient absorption problems and can cause leaky gut.[44]

Some other things that can cause irritation of the gut include GMOs, vaccines and stress.

Glyphosate

Glyphosate is another thing we all should be concerned about today. Glyphosate is the vital ingredient found in the herbicide Roundup, which is used world-wide as a weed killer for crops. Recent studies and research show that glyphosate poses a significant health concern for the general public. In fact, according to a recent study on rats, it has been linked to gene disruption and sexual development. It also can cause interference with beneficial bacteria in the gut, leading to bad microbes taking over and wreaking havoc.[45]

Other studies suggest that glyphosate is a contributor to the rise in chronic disease, especially in the Western world. Many food products today are made with genetically modified corn, soy, wheat and sugar beets and a large number of them contain traces of glyphosate.[46] Alarmingly, many processed foods are now being contaminated, especially cereals. Another disturbing fact regarding glyphosate is that it binds vital nutrients your body needs including iron, zinc, manganese and more to the soil. In other words, it prevents crops from absorbing them, so in turn we're not receiving the benefits we used to from various plants.[47] If you are concerned about glyphosate in your food, make sure you look for products that are marked non GMO to help avoid it.

Ways To Build A Healthy Gut

The good news is that there are a variety of ways to keep your gut healthy, including paying attention to what you eat and consume. Following are some ways to nourish and heal your body and keep it functioning at an optimal level.

1. *Eliminate Foods with Added Sugar*—While many people love sugar, it is actually considered a toxin by many nutrition experts and the cause of many diseases. It's a proven fact that sugar causes inflammation and changes the balance of good and bad bacteria in your gut and also contributes to yeast over-growth. Those who consume a lot of sugar have a higher level of bad bacteria, so it is best to limit sugary foods in your diet and enjoy them more as an occasional treat. Eating a diet rich in whole foods, especially vegetables, is a better, healthier way to keep your gut balanced.
2. *Eat Plenty of Whole Foods*—Eating plenty of whole grains, nuts and vegetables is important for keeping your gut healthy. Whole grains and veggies not only contain fiber to keep things moving, but also

feed the good bacteria in your gut. Make sure you look for fresh whole foods that are in season and include them in your meals and snacking.

3. ***Add Fruit to Your Diet***—While it is important to include more fruit and vegetables in your diet, it is important not to go way overboard with fruit. Fruit contains a variety of nutrients and antioxidants, yet also contains natural sugars that may have an effect on your microbiome. If you enjoy eating fruit, you may want to limit your fruit consumption to 2-3 servings per day, while working to heal your gut. You can also choose those fruits that have lower sugar content. For example, strawberries, blueberries and blackberries have lower sugar content than a mango or pineapple.

4. ***Add More Fermented Foods to Your Diet***—Fermented foods are rich in probiotics, which help keep your gut healthy and bacteria in check. Probiotic foods such as sauerkraut, pickles, kefir, yogurt and tempeh work to balance the gut. Try including more fermented foods to your meals or snacks to reap their benefits and keep your gut healthy.

5. ***Watch the Caffeine***—While caffeine is often considered a pick me up and may give you a boost of energy, it can also bring you down and leave you feeling ill if you consume too much. Coffee and other caffeine drinks are acidic and can cause stomach irritability and promote bad bacteria overgrowth. In turn, over consumption, along with other unhealthy eating habits may contribute to leaky gut, auto immune disease and other illnesses.

6. ***Eat More Anti-Inflammatory Foods***—If your gut is inflamed and causing pain, discomfort or absorption problems, you need to calm the storm. One of the best things you can do for your gut is to choose more foods that fight inflammation. The good news is there are many anti-inflammatory foods and some of the best ones include fresh fruit and vegetables. Fruit contains essential vitamins, minerals and anti-oxidants your body needs to heal and operate at an optimal level. Try adding more berries, oranges, grapes and cherries to your diet. Berries and cherries are a super food and help fight inflammation, as well as strengthen the immune system. (See Chapter 4: Eating for Iron

Deficiency for more information.)

7. *Avoid Processed Foods*—Processed foods typically contain large amounts of trans-fats, sodium, sugar and high fructose corn syrup. Many processed foods are also loaded with chemicals, preservatives and artificial sweeteners, all of which wreak havoc on your gut and create an imbalance in your gut flora. Consumers often buy processed foods because they are convenient to make and cheap to buy. In addition, there are thousands of choices making them appealing to many individuals. A better option is to choose more whole foods, particularly vegetables. Greens and cruciferous vegetables are extremely healing for the gut. Both contain antioxidants, phytochemicals and have a variety of vitamins and minerals that nourish and help heal the body. They also may help prevent the colonization of unhealthy bacteria in the gut, including Helicobacter pylori (H pylori) and other organisms. When buying any processed foods, make sure you read the food label and avoid those products with long ingredient lists. Your best bet is to always shoot for 5 ingredients or less. (See Chapter 4: Eating for Iron Deficiency.)

8. *Add Bone Broth to Your Diet*—Drinking bone broth is a great way to help nourish and heal your gut. Bone broth is rich in nutrients and vitamins that help reduce inflammation in the body and is especially beneficial for the gut. Some vitamins found in bone broth include zinc, vitamin A and vitamin K. It also contains iron, which is beneficial for those with iron deficiency. Additionally, bone broth contains collagen and amino acids that help heal and seal the gut lining. Many people enjoy the medicinal effects of bone broth, as well as the comforting feeling it provides.

9. *Eat More Good Fats*—When it comes to adding fat into our diet, many people are confused, and rightly so! There's a lot of conflicting information out there in regard to fat, and many people don't know what to believe. These days, you can find people who try and limit their fat intake and others who are trying to load up on it (think Keto Diet or Atkins Diet). Still others are stuck on the low-fat craze idea from the 90s and stock up on low-fat foods. Eating a healthy diet rich

in nutrients and fat is important for overall health. Limiting fat in your diet is not a good idea and can have serious side effects on your body. Restricting fat can disrupt your hormones, impair digestion, weaken your bones and muscles, affect your kidneys and compromise your immune system. Our bodies need fat to function properly and perform peak functions. Try adding more healthy fat foods to your diet such as avocados, nuts, seeds, coconut oil and olives to keep your gut healthy.

10. *Take a Good Probiotic*—Along with eating a healthy diet of whole foods, taking a probiotic supplement will help balance the good bacteria in your gut. Many people today eat the wrong types of food, and are exposed to toxins in the home and environment. Many people also use products on their skin that can disrupt the bacteria in the body. These imbalances often create unhealthy gut flora. That is why it is important to take a probiotic supplement to help populate the good bacteria in your gut.

11. *Reduce Stress*—Chronic stress and anxiety can be hard on your body and may have an affect on your stomach. Make sure you are scheduling time in your day for yourself. Take some time to relax and enjoy yourself. Taking a walk outside can be very beneficial. Yoga, meditation, reading and prayer can also be calming and helpful. It is also important to schedule time for fun. Why not plan on meeting a friend for dinner, go to a movie or concert, or go have a massage or pedicure? There are many options.

12. *Add Cod Liver Oil to Your Diet*—Studies show that cod liver oil is quite useful for healing the gut. Cod liver oil is rich in vitamin A, vitamin D and omega 3 fatty acids your body needs to thrive. It is also highly anti-inflammatory. Try adding a teaspoon of cod liver oil to your daily diet to benefit from its healing properties.

13. *Take a Zinc Supplement*—Many people are deficient in zinc and aren't aware they have an issue. Unfortunately if you are not getting enough zinc in your diet, it can cause a variety of problems including poor immunity, thinning hair and leaky gut. Studies show that taking a zinc supplement can help tighten the gut wall and help alleviate

permeability issues. Try adding a zinc supplement to your diet to help strengthen your immunity and your gut.

14. **Brush and Floss Your Teeth**—While you might wonder how brushing and flossing your teeth can affect your gut, there is a correlation. In fact, studies show that bacteria found in your mouth can actually make its way to your stomach and cause problems that lead to ill health. Make sure you pay attention to your oral hygiene.

Wholey Cow Affirmations:

I release any pain or discomfort I may have.
I send love and gratitude to my stomach and inner being.

CHAPTER 6

I Am Ironman?
Exercise and Iron Deficiency

"We do not stop exercising because we grow old – We grow old because we stop exercising."
—Kenneth Cooper

Listen To Your Body

While everyone needs to stay active, exercise can be tough when your body is run down and fatigued from low iron. Many people suffering with iron deficiency have a hard time getting off the coach or out of bed some days, let alone going for a walk or heading to the gym. Even if you are person who is used to being active, ran marathons or competed in ironman triathlons, if you have an iron deficiency it's time to listen to your body. Your body needs time to rest and recover when your iron is low. This may be hard for some individuals, especially if you are an active person, but rest is important.

As you begin feeling better from iron supplementation and eating more iron-rich foods, it is a good idea to start adding some activity to your day.

It's important to start out slow. Try going for a short walk outside to get some fresh air. You can also try doing some stretches at home or some yoga poses to get some blood flowing and your muscles moving. If you're ok doing these things, you can take a longer walk, add in more stretches, try a yoga class or something else.

Rest As Needed

As you start to gain more energy, it is ok to venture out to the gym if this is your thing and you are feeling up to it. Make sure you stick to a low intensity workout to start instead of running or doing a high intensity workout. Moreover, make sure you shorten up your regular routine and stop if you feel winded or short of breath. If you feel better after catching your breath for a few minutes, it is probably alright to continue. Otherwise, there is nothing wrong with calling it a day and trying again tomorrow. As you continue to feel better, feel free to add to your gym routine or other work out plan. Additionally, you may want to have some sort of iron-rich snack before you exercise to give you a boost of energy. It is also a good idea to have a snack after exercising to help re-fuel your body and iron stores. Try eating a handful of nuts, having a smoothie, eating a banana with some peanut butter or some other iron-rich snack you enjoy. (See Chapter 4: Eating for Iron Deficiency for other snack ideas.)

Timing is Everything

Remember—it is always best to work out when you feel the most energized. For some people that may be in the morning after a good night's rest and a good breakfast filled with iron-rich foods. For others, it may be later on in the day or maybe after work. Everyone is different, so exercise when it feels best for your body and works with your schedule.

Keep a Positive Mind-Set about Exercise

If you are person who doesn't exercise on a regular basis or at all, you may want to change your mind-set about exercise. Exercise not only is good for your body, but is also good for your mind and spirit. That's right! Exercise has more benefits than just helping you lose weight and stay fit. It can relieve stress, make you feel more alive and alert and help you focus more. Granted, when you are sick and your body is run down, exercise may be the furthest thing from your mind. However, if your body is healing and you want to live a healthy lifestyle, exercise can have a lot of benefits, some of which I've listed below.

Immediate Effects on The Brain
Exercise causes immediate effects on the brain by increasing the neurotransmitters dopamine and serotonin, which make you feel good (e.g., think of a runner's high). It also helps improve your reaction times.

> **ARE YOU AWARE?**
> Exercise can boost your mood, improve your memory and give you more energy.

Improves Attention and Long-Term Memory
Exercise helps improve your attention, which can help with brain fog and long-term memory.

Long Lasting Effects of Good Mood
Exercise promotes long lasting effects for your body and can help make your brain stronger and function better.[48]

How to Reap the Benefits of Exercise
There are many ways to reap the benefits of exercise and it all starts with making a commitment and taking an initiative. Some ways to feel the benefits of exercise include:

Consistency
While it is ideal to exercise every day, make sure you shoot for 3-4 times per week. Again, if you are not feeling up to it, or have a low energy day, listen to your body and take time to rest. Consistency, however, does matter. Try to develop a routine, as you will be more apt to make exercise part of your schedule. This way if you miss a day for some reason, you'll be more likely to get back at it.

Get Your Heart Rate Up

It's important to get your heart rate up when you are feeling better to take advantage of those feel-good hormones from exercising. Exercise helps clear your head and boosts your mood. It is also good for your heart, so it's important to incorporate some sort of aerobic exercise in your routine.

If you have issues with your heart or other medical concerns, make sure to consult your doctor.

Make it Worthwhile

To reap the full benefits of exercise, make sure you exercise and stay active for at least 30 minutes at a time or longer. This should allow enough time to get an energy boost, as well as strengthen your heart, mind and muscles. Again, talk to your doctor if you have any concerns about exercising and your health.

Make Exercise Fun

Exercise can be fun and exhilarating and can help make you feel more alive physically. If you find yourself making excuses not to exercise, you might need to change your mind-set about exercise. If you are a person who doesn't necessarily like running, going to the gym or walking, that's ok—there are plenty of other activities you can try.

I personally love to exercise and incorporate a variety of activities into my routine. I walk daily. I also enjoy biking, yoga, weight training and playing tennis. You can also find me hula hooping and jumping on my trampoline from time to time. In fact, I have a full size trampoline in my yard, which I use through the spring and fall seasons. In addition, I have a mini rebounder trampoline in my basement I jump on in the winter months. There's just something about jumping that makes me come alive. It always puts a smile on my face and makes me happy.

Many people get stuck on focusing what they don't like, instead of thinking about activities they might enjoy. If you can't think of anything, why not focus on some activities you liked to do as a child? I am sure you can find some activity from your childhood that makes you happy! Why not dance, skip, jump rope, swing or play basketball to get your happy on? The point is to find some form of exercise you enjoy and stay active. If you have questions or concerns, make sure you consult your doctor about where to start.

Wholey Cow Affirmations:

I am getting stronger every day.
My blood is healthy and energizes my body.

CHAPTER 7

Dealing With The Symptoms

"Action is the foundational key to all success."
—Pablo Picasso

Rise and Shine?

While the vast majority of people feel refreshed and rejuvenated after a good night's sleep, those who suffer with chronic low iron often wake up tired regardless of how much sleep they may have had. For many people with iron deficiency, it is common to feel sleepy, lethargy or not think clearly when waking. It's no wonder some individuals may not feel like getting out of bed. I remember the groggy feeling and fog that surrounded my head quite vividly. I wanted nothing more than to escape from the haze and get some energy going. Fortunately there are some things you can try to get your day going and boost your energy.

Eat Breakfast

One of the most important things you can do to get your day going and to feel less groggy is to eat a good breakfast that includes plenty of iron-rich food. After a long night's rest, your body needs fuel to re-energize itself. Make sure you take some time to eat some healthy food. Breakfast doesn't have to be hard or complicated. If you are in a hurry, why not have a banana and peanut butter? You can grab a granola bar, nuts or an apple to take with you and eat on the way. If you have time, why not try making some eggs? Try adding in some greens, onions, spinach, tomatoes or other vegetables to boost your iron intake. You can also have some other protein along with your eggs such as ham, sausage, bacon or some left-over chicken from the last night's dinner. Adding some sort of meat will also help boost your iron intake. There are many options to add iron to your eggs or other breakfast foods. You can also try making a smoothie. Many brands of protein powder have a high iron content, so they make an excellent breakfast option because they provide a decent way to get a generous boost of iron to start your day. Make sure you look for a high-quality protein powder, preferably an organic version, or one that incorporates a lot of healthy ingredients and has low or no sugar. Make sure you pay attention to the food labels to learn what's included in the product before purchasing.

Smoothies became my go-to breakfast when my ferritin levels were super low and I still make them almost daily. Smoothies provide a good dose of morning protein and iron, especially after adding in greens, fruit and a few super foods. Most mornings I have a smoothie for breakfast along with a slice of ham, piece of bacon or some other meat. A few hours later I typically grab a handful of nuts, trail mix or dried apricots for a snack.

Eating this way helped me alleviate some early morning brain fog, although the affect was not always immediate. It takes a little time for your body to process both the food and iron. Keep in mind that there are many options for eating an iron-rich breakfast. (See Chapter 4: Eating For Iron Deficiency for more ideas for eating healthy.)

Tea Time
Another thing that helped me get my day going was drinking a cup of tea. I know some people are concerned about the tannins in tea and their effect on iron absorption, but early on, I really needed some caffeine to

function and help me stay awake. My iron was going up with supplementing and eating more iron rich foods, so I didn't let it bother me. Remember, we are all unique individuals and what works for one, may not work for another. If you are concerned about absorption issues, you can always wait an hour or two after taking your supplements and eating to have your cup of tea. You could also just have a cup of tea with your meal and not worry about it. Your body will let you know if there is a problem. (See Chapter 4: Eating For Iron Deficiency for more about iron absorption inhibitors.)

Caffeinated Tea

There are many options when it comes to tea. My favorite happens to be chai tea, which I like to sweeten with a bit of stevia. Green tea is another great option that I also enjoy and have from time to time. Green tea has many medicinal properties and can help give you a boost of energy in the morning or afternoon. There are many other caffeinated varieties that may help you get through your day.

Herbal Tea

If you want to avoid caffeine, there are plenty of herbal teas you may like and find uplifting. Some herbal teas, such as chamomile, peppermint or lemon balm have calming effects that may help with anxiety or irritability. Other herbal varieties may be anti-inflammatory, boost immunity or help stimulate brain function. You might want to investigate ginger, turmeric, licorice or ginseng as options to try.

Red raspberry leaf tea has been used throughout the ages and is known for its healing properties. Red raspberry leaf tea is high in nutrients, antioxidants and is anti-inflammatory. Some nutrients found in red raspberry leaf tea include B vitamins and iron, which are especially beneficial to those suffering with iron deficiency. Some other nutrients found in red raspberry leaf tea include calcium, magnesium, vitamin E and potassium. In addition, red raspberry leaf tea is high in vitamin C, which helps build immunity and may help with iron absorption. Red raspberry leaf tea is also beneficial for digestion. Moreover, red raspberry leaf tea helps balance hormones, which may be helpful for women who suffer with heavy periods. It can also be beneficial for pregnant women, as it helps strengthen the uterus and pelvic muscles and may make labor easier for some women.[49]

There are many other varieties of tea that have medicinal properties, so you may want to do some investigating on your own to find one that suits your particular needs.

Oil Up

Using essential oils is something else you might want to try to help ease some symptoms you may be experiencing. While there are over 100 different commonly used essential oils, I found a number of them beneficial for iron deficiency. If you are not familiar with essential oils, they are natural oils that are extracted from various plant species and are used for a variety of medicinal purposes. Essential oils have been used for centuries and date back to biblical times. Many essential oils have therapeutic effects and can be used for a variety of ailments. Some oils can also be used for perfume and are popular because of their aromatic properties. Essential oils typically come from the flower, stem, root, leaves or fruit of various plants. There are a variety of application methods for essential oils including topical application and diffusion. Some oils can also be taken orally. If you are interested in using essential oils, make sure you choose a therapeutic-grade oil and read up on the safest and best application methods.

Lemon Oil

Lemon essential oil is a universal oil that has many health benefits. It is loaded with vitamin C, which can help build immunity and help treat a cold. It has also been shown to help with anxiety, arthritis, fatigue, stress and more. Lemon oil in particular helps stimulate the production of red and white blood cells and may help with the absorption of iron supplements.[50] The scent of lemon oil is also uplifting and helps promote positive energy.

> **ARE YOU AWARE?**
>
> *Lemon oil in particular helps stimulate the production of red and white blood cells and may help with the absorption of iron supplements.*

One way I helped get my energy up in the morning was to add a drop of lemon essential oil to my morning glass of water. It helped clear my head and get rid of my brain fog. Additionally, it helped ease some of the fatigue and memory issues I was having. Although some sources say not to take any essential oils internally, others disagree.

Lemon oil can also be diffused, inhaled, added to bath water or applied topically. Make sure you use a carrier oil if you choose to apply lemon oil to your skin to avoid any skin sensitivity.

Note: If you choose to add a drop of lemon oil to your drinking water, make sure you are using a therapeutic-grade oil and one marked as a dietary or vitality supplement.

Other Citrus Oils

Other citrus oils, such as grapefruit, orange, lime or tangerine can also help promote iron absorption and may help alleviate fatigue. These citrus oils are rich in vitamin C, which help build immunity. In addition, they may help in the absorption of both iron-rich foods and supplements. Make sure you choose a therapeutic-grade oil and read up on safety, dietary oils and best application methods.

Clary Sage

Clary sage is medicinal oil that is often used to help balance hormones. Many women find clary sage oil beneficial for cramps, PMS, bloating and hot flashes. Clary sage is antispasmodic, so it helps relax the muscles and nerves. Additionally, some women have found that clary sage helps ease heavy menstrual cycles, which is a common cause of iron deficiency among women, especially during perimenopause.

The affects may not be immediate, as it takes some time to get your body back in balance, but it does work for many women. If you want to give clary sage essential oil a try, make sure you use it every month consistently. I applied clary sage oil to my lower abdomen daily for the 2 weeks prior to my cycle. You can also use a carrier oil, such as coconut oil, almond oil, jojoba oil or olive oil to dilute the oil to aid in absorption.

Clary sage is also beneficial for anxiety and is a great stress reliever. Moreover, it helps relieve insomnia, promotes skin health and may be beneficial for blood circulation.

Note: If you have questions or concerns about using clary sage essential oil, make sure you talk with your doctor, naturopath, acupuncturist or other qualified professional.

Frankincense

Frankincense is a sacred oil and has been around for thousands of years. Most people are familiar with frankincense, as it is mentioned throughout the bible and in particular in the story of the Three Wise Men bearing gifts of gold, frankincense and myrrh for the baby Jesus. Frankincense has many health benefits, so it's no surprise it has been treasured for centuries. Frankincense comes from the boswellia tree native to Africa, India and parts of Arabia and has an earthy or woodsy smell. In ancient times, people used frankincense resin for incense or perfume, as it helps induce a feeling of peace and tranquility and helps relieve stress. They also used frankincense for healing salves, anointing and a variety of other ailments.

Frankincense is a powerful oil that has many other healing properties including its ability to boost immunity, help prevent infections and help prevent cancer. Frankincense also is antiseptic in nature and is known for its anti-aging properties. Additionally frankincense may help regulate menstruation in women.[51]

I use frankincense oil daily and find it very grounding. I like to apply a drop or two on my face along with my morning moisturizer. It helps instill a calm feeling, as well as promotes healthy skin. You can also apply frankincense to your abdomen or other areas of your skin or diffuse it in the air to help promote a peaceful environment or to help relieve anxiety or stress.

Lavender

Lavender is one of the most popular essential oils available and it's easy to see why. Lavender has many health benefits and its soft, light scent is calming and balancing. Lavender oil is anti-inflammatory, anti-microbial and contains anti-bacterial properties. It's not surprising lavender has been used for its medicinal affects since ancient times. Lavender is a universal oil that is often used for its uplifting aromatic properties and can be used for the treatment of minor aches and pains, as well as wound healing. Some studies suggest that lavender essential oil's calming properties may be beneficial to those suffering from anxiety, Alzheimer's and other illnesses. Many people like to use lavender oil to help relieve stress and boost their mood. Lavender essential oil can also be used to heal bruises, minor cuts and scrapes.

Lavender oil happens to be one of my favorite essential oils. I love the smell and find it very uplifting and soothing. I have used lavender oil for years, but found it particularly calming for days when I felt anxious or had an uneasy feeling. I like to apply lavender to my wrists or temples and sometimes just inhale some of the fumes from the bottle. You can also diffuse lavender in your bedroom, office or bathroom to help create a peaceful, calm environment. Additionally, you can add a few drops of lavender to your bath to you help you unwind. You can also put a few drops on your pillow to help you have a restful nights sleep.

Geranium
Geranium essential oil is another oil that can help balance hormones. Many women find that geranium oil helps with PMS, hot flashes and irritability. Geranium oil has a sweet scent that many people find uplifting. It also has a variety of therapeutic properties and can be used as both an antidepressant and antiseptic. Geranium oil can be used to boost your mood, help alleviate anxiety and help fight fatigue. In addition, geranium oil contains properties that promote radiant skin and may help reduce fine lines and wrinkles. It can also be used to treat acne.

Although I like the smell of geranium, it is not an oil I use every day, as I prefer some other oils over it. I do use geranium oil occasionally to uplift my spirits if I am feeling a little out of sorts. I also use geranium to help balance my hormones and obtain a normal cycle. You can apply geranium oil to your lower abdomen or forearms along with a carrier oil, such as coconut oil or jojoba oil. You can also add a few drops of geranium oil to a diffuser to breathe in its fresh scent to help boost your mood. Additionally, adding a few drops of geranium oil to your bath may help alleviate anxiety and promote a sense of peace.

Valor
Valor is a popular oil blend that is very powerful and restorative. It is known for its ability to help boost courage and confidence, as it helps restore physical, mental and emotional energies. Valor oil is comprised of a variety of oils including black spruce, blue tansy, geranium, frankincense and camphor wood. This oil blend happens to be one of my favorite oils. I use it daily to help keep stress at bay and instill positivity and self-assurance.

Valor has many health benefits as it is anti-inflammatory, anti-viral, anti-bacterial and has properties that help inhibit anxiety. Valor also helps boost energy, helps relieve stress and helps boost immunity, so it may be particularly useful for those dealing with symptoms of iron deficiency

I like to apply a drop or two to the back of my neck in the morning to instill a positive tone for the day and alleviate any anxious thoughts. Besides that, I typically carry this oil in my purse and apply it whenever I want a little boost of confidence or boost of energy. You can also apply valor to your wrists or temples or diffuse the oil to create a calm, peaceful atmosphere.

Vetiver
Vetiver essential oil has been used since ancient times and has a variety of medicinal properties. Vetiver is popular in Ayurvedic medicine and also considered a sacred herb. Vetiver is a perennial grass that is native to India and has an earthy or woody smell. When distilled, vetiver oil is rich in antioxidants, making it a prized oil. Vetiver also has antiseptic properties and is useful in the reduction of infections and killing bacteria. Vetiver oil also has anti-aging properties that help prevent wrinkles and help reduce scarring and acne. In addition, vetiver oil is a very grounding oil and is known for its ability to soothe, comfort and create a sense of peace and calm.

I used vetiver oil when my anxiety level was high and I felt extremely agitated and worried. Vetiver is a powerful oil and its calming effects can be felt almost immediately after applying it to the back of your neck. In my experience, it seems to take the edge off more than any other oil and provides a sense of comfort. It's not surprising vetiver oil has been shown as an effective treatment for ADHD and anxiety in various studies.

Vetiver oil can be used in a number of different ways. You can apply a drop or two on your wrists, neck, feet or chest area. You can also diffuse vetiver oil in a room, or add 5-10 drops in a hot bath.

Ylang Ylang

Ylang ylang essential oil has a sweet, floral scent that is uplifting and energizing and has been prized for its medicinal properties for centuries. Ylang ylang oil comes from the flowers of the ylang ylang tree, which are found in plush tropical areas in the South Pacific such as Ecuador, Indonesia and the Philippines. Ylang ylang oil is rich in antioxidants and contains anti-inflammatory properties that can help ease a variety of discomforts. Ylang ylang has other health benefits too, including helping to improve blood flow and antiseptic properties. It is also known as an aphrodisiac and has been shown to be an effective antidepressant and sedative.

Not everyone likes the smell of ylang ylang oil, but I love it and find it cheery. I like to apply it to my wrists or heart area when I need a boost of energy or want to uplift my spirits. Sometimes I apply a drop of ylang ylang oil along with grapefruit oil to the back of my neck for an additional pick me up. Ylang ylang is a good oil to try if you are feeling a little anxious, run down or just have an uneasy feeling you want to get rid of. You can also diffuse ylang ylang oil in a room to help elevate your mood. Moreover, you can add a few drops of ylang ylang to your bath if you want to unwind before bed and promote a restful night's sleep.

Calming the Cold

Many people who are iron deficient have trouble keeping warm. Iron is needed to oxygenate your blood, and when you don't have enough iron to transport oxygen throughout your body, you can be left with a cold feeling. Since your hands and feet are further away than some other organs, they are most affected. They can feel cold to the touch and may turn red or purple in color. Unfortunately, when your hands and feet are cold, many people tend to feel cold all over. Some individuals feel colder at night, which was the case for me. In fact, when my iron stores were super low, I remember going to bed wearing lots of layers (pajamas, sweatshirt, socks and hand gloves) and using an extra blanket. After several hours, I usually was able to warm up a bit and remove some layers.

If you have issues staying warm, thankfully there are some things you can try to help get through it.

Take a Bath
Hot baths are not only soothing and comforting, but can warm your whole body. Try taking a bath before bed so your body doesn't feel so chilled. When your body is warmed up from a bath, you may find it easier to fall asleep and more apt to get a good night's rest.

Wear Gloves
If your hands are constantly cold, you may want to find yourself a pair of light weight gloves you can wear around the house or at work. I have several pairs of knit half gloves (fingers tips exposed) that I wear around my house to help keep my hands warm. My husband likes to call them "house gloves" and sometimes reminds me put them on. I forget sometimes how cold my hands can feel to the touch and need a reminder. I used to have a pair of gloves I'd keep in my desk drawer at work too. They may look a little odd or funny, but they do help keep your hands warm. Holding a cup of tea or coffee in your hands can be helpful as well.

Wear Wool Socks/Slippers
If you tend to have cold feet, especially at night, you may want to invest in some warm wool socks or slipper socks you can wear around the house or to bed. I always wear slippers around the house to help keep my feet warm. I also wore socks to bed consistently when my iron stores were super low and still wear them periodically to help keep my feet warm in the winter months. They do help, but I sometimes find them lying on the floor in morning, which is actually a good thing.

Pile On the Blankets

If you are super cold at night, you may want to add an extra blanket to your bed to help keep you warm. I have an extra blanket on my coach too, which I use a lot when I am reading or watching TV. I have grown to love blankets. I find them comforting and enjoy snuggling up with them. Make sure you invest in some extra blankets to help you stay warm.

Drink a Glass of Red Wine

Some people reach for a glass of red wine when they are cold. That's not surprising as red wine contains tannins and histamines that have warming properties that help warm the body. Alcohol dilates your blood vessels and increases blood flow, which may help you feel warm. Many people notice their hands and feet feel warmer after drinking a glass of wine. Keep in mind that while red wine may help warm your body, it may have an effect iron absorption because of the tannins.

Cozy Up To a Fire

There's nothing like a hot fire to help you warm up. Fires can be relaxing and help create a cozy environment. I like to sit in front of my fireplace with a hot cup of tea, warm blanket and a good book. Fires can also be calming if you just sit and stare at the fire and bask in the heat. If you have a fireplace, you may want to consider spending more time sitting in front of it to both relax and warm your body.

Sauna/Hot Tub

Sitting in a sauna or hot tub can also help warm your body. Both can be relaxing and help warm your core. If you have a sauna or hot tub at home, you may want to indulge in it more often to help you stay warm. Some exercise clubs or gyms may also have saunas or hot tubs you can use. Perhaps you can set aside a day or time to enjoy some extra heat and relaxation.

Hot Yoga

If you currently take yoga classes or you're interested in trying yoga, hot yoga can definitely help you warm up. Obviously hot yoga is not something you would want to try if your iron is super low or you are extremely fatigued from low iron, but it may be something you want to investigate or try down the road when you are feeling better and have more energy. Hot yoga consists of a series of yoga poses done in a room heated to a very warm temperature (often to 105°F). There are other styles that may be done at somewhat lower temps, but Bikram yoga is probably the most popular. Hot yoga can be invigorating and warms you from the core. I sometimes do a hot yoga class when I am feeling chilled and want some deep stretching.

Acupuncture

Acupuncture is another great alternative option to try for the treatment of iron deficiency. Personally, I've found acupuncture to be quite beneficial. Acupuncture has been used for centuries to treat anemia and symptoms of tiredness, weakness and more. In fact, studies show that acupuncture can help bring up ferritin levels, as well as help lower your total iron binding capacity (TIBC). It can also help improve spleen function, which helps process food and aids in the iron absorption process.[52] Often times, acupuncture is used in conjunction with Chinese herbs to build and nourish the blood.

I chose to work with an acupuncturist because I wanted to find a natural way to deal with the problems I was having. Like many other women, I suffered with heavy periods for years. I never thought too much about it, until it literally drained the life out of me over time. When I figured out what was wrong, I visited my gynecologist. Besides prescribing iron supplements and changing my diet to include more iron-rich foods, she also gave me several options to treat the heavy bleeding I was experiencing. Taking birth control or having an invasive procedure, however, just didn't sit well with me. I am more of a natural girl and alternative care was much more appealing to me. I opted to give acupuncture a try instead. While the affects weren't immediate, I am happy to say that the treatments, along with the prescribed herbs my acupuncturist recommended, helped me to regain my balance. They also helped ease some of the fatigue and tiredness I was experiencing and helped increase my energy levels. I am very blessed and grateful for having the opportunity to work with an acupuncturist and highly recommend it. Some women, however, have positive results with western medicine practices and are happy with their decisions. Again, keep in mind that everyone is different and each situation is unique, so it's always best to do what feels right for you.

Calming Your Mind and Thoughts

Many people who have iron deficiency suffer with anxiety and it's not fun. The good news is there are a variety of natural remedies you can try to help relieve some of the uneasiness, worry and out-of-balance feelings you may be dealing with. I already mentioned some teas you might want to try, as well as a number of essential oils to get some relief, but there are a few other things you might find helpful to calm your mind and thoughts.

L-theanine

L-theanine is a supplement that I found useful to relieve some anxiety symptoms. L-theanine is an amino acid found in green tea and black tea and some varieties of mushrooms. When ingested, it affects certain chemicals in the brain including dopamine and serotonin, which can affect your mood, sleep and emotions. L-theanine has calming properties that help relieve stress, anxiety and help promote relaxation and restful sleep. Moreover, studies show that L-theanine may help increase cognitive functions and improve attention. While you can drink tea to get some effects of L-theanine, it is also available in capsule form, which you can find in some grocery stores, drug stores and online. L-theanine is generally considered safe to use. Check with your doctor if you have any questions or concerns before taking the supplement.[53]

Gaba

Gaba is another supplement that can be useful for symptoms of anxiety. Like many other people, I had never heard of gaba before I developed iron deficiency, but I learned of it from a chiropractic doctor. Gaba is short for gamma aminobutyric acid, which is neurotransmitter that helps send messages from the brain to your nervous system. Gaba has calming effects on the body and has been shown to help ease anxiety, stress and depression. It has also been shown to enhance mood, help with insomnia and decrease inflammation in the body. Gaba is considered safe to use for most individuals, but make sure you check with your doctor if you have questions or concerns, as it may interact with other medications or supplements. Additionally, it is not recommended for pregnant women, or those nursing.

Meditation/Yoga
Meditation is another thing you can try if you are dealing with anxiety or having trouble relaxing. Meditation helps calm the mind and thoughts. Since many people who suffer with iron deficiency experience worry and unease, sitting still may be the furthest thing from their mind. Meditation naturally helps ease tension and promotes an overall sense of well-being. It also helps you re-connect to your true self. For many individuals, meditation is peaceful and can be a form of spirituality and way to connect with God and a higher power.

If you are a beginner, it is best to start out slow. Many people have a hard time trying to still their mind. This is understandable, as thoughts often race by and can take us places we don't necessarily want to go. If you are having difficulty, don't worry. It takes a great deal of practice to focus on the present moment. Start out by sitting silently for a few minutes and build from there. If your mind starts to wander, just begin again. Over time you will be able to sit quietly longer and enjoy the peace and comfort it brings. You can also try just repeating the word "peace" or some other word or mantra that instills a sense of peace and calm to help you find a place of comfort.

If meditation isn't your thing, you can also try yoga or some other meditative practice. Yoga is calming and can help you stay in balance. Many people find yoga relaxing and peaceful. Many yoga poses are restorative in nature and can also be invigorating. When you practice yoga, you create a flow of energy that can uplift both your mood and spirit. Many people feel refreshed and a sense calm after participating in a yoga class.

I personally love practicing yoga and always feel better after finishing a yoga class. In addition, I like to sit quietly in nature and always enjoy a morning meditative walk. These practices help to relieve stress, help me stay inspired and keep me in balance.

Affirmations

Practicing affirmations is another way to help relieve the stress and anxiety that can go along with iron deficiency and anemia. It is easy to get caught up in negative thoughts and emotions when you are not feeling well, fatigued or agitated. The problem with negative thoughts, however, is that they can escalate into more and more. The next thing you know you can have a pity party going on, which unfortunately can drag you down even further and can make matters worse. It can also affect your relationships, work and more. The good news is that turning your thoughts and emotions into something positive can also have the same affect and can be quite powerful. I know this can be easier said than done, but practicing positive affirmations has been shown to be a useful tool for healing. In fact, studies show that using affirmations can ease stress, boost self-esteem, help with depression, improve confidence and more.[54]

If you are not familiar with affirmations, they are positive statements that can help you overcome negative thinking and can help change your thought patterns. When you repeat something consistently, you will start to believe it, and that is where change and healing takes place. Your mind believes what you're telling it and your body naturally responds in a positive way.

If you are wondering how to use affirmations, it's pretty easy. It's really a matter of turning something around from negative to positive. For example, instead of telling yourself, "I am so tired," when you are feeling fatigued, try saying, "I give my body permission to rest and heal. I am getting better every day." This gives your negative thought a different spin and helps alleviate added stress and anxiety. It also helps eliminate additional negativity. Moreover, it sends your body feel-good vibes, which promote healing.

There are many ways you can use affirmations in your life and the more you use them, the easier they become. I have listed a number of affirmations throughout the book you can use. You can also find plenty of positive affirmations online, purchase an affirmation book or look on Pinterest or other websites for affirmations to use. There are many options. I've included space at the end of this book for you to create some of your own affirmations. Remember—affirmations don't have to be hard or complicated. Just focus on saying something positive and uplifting. I guarantee with a little practice, you will find them useful.

Self-Care

Many people are good at taking care of others, but not always good at taking care of themselves. When your body is run down and fatigued from too little iron, a little self-care is probably just what you need to feel better. Giving yourself time to rest is important and a big part of the healing process. You don't necessarily have to go to bed, but there is nothing wrong with taking a nap.

There are quite a number of other ways you can practice self-care. It can be as simple as doing something you like or enjoy, such as going to a movie or buying yourself a cup of coffee. If you are too tired to go out, why not find a good movie on Netflix or make a good cup of tea? You can also treat yourself to some good dark chocolate or maybe have a glass of wine. If you like to read, why not take some time to read a good book or magazine? If you fall asleep in the process, that's ok. It's good for your body.

If you are feeling run down or achy, you might want to treat yourself to a pedicure or massage. These services can be rejuvenating and help you escape from any anxious thoughts you might be feeling. They can also boost your mood and self-esteem. You can also take a warm bath to help you relax and ease any fatigue you might be experiencing. Try adding some essentials oils to your bath water such as lavender, geranium or clary sage to help uplift your spirits and calm your mind.

As you begin to feel better and more energetic, you might want to go shopping, take in a concert or go on a nature walk. There are many possibilities. The point is to start incorporating more things in your day that bring you joy.

Healthy Relationships

Dealing with the symptoms of iron deficiency is not always easy and can take a toll on you and the people around you, especially family members. Many people may not understand what you might be going through and may have a hard time relating to your problems and symptoms, especially if overall you appear to be fine. Not feeling supported by those around you can be a big problem. If you are dealing with iron deficiency, do not forget that the vast majority of people are uneducated on the ailment and may not be able to relate to what you are going through and experiencing. I know from experience that this can be very frustrating and make you feel very alone. It can also bring about emotions like anger, sorrow and resentment. Many people may also feel unloved or disrespected. If your family and friends don't understand some of your symptoms, or why you may not appear to be the person you used to be, take heart. There are others out there who are going through the same experience.

The good news is there are people out there who can help. Some people may turn to counseling, but there are a variety of support groups available as well. People you meet in support groups can more easily relate, offer advice and provide helpful information and support. I found a number of Facebook groups set up specifically for those suffering with iron deficiency and iron deficiency anemia, which I found extremely helpful. It is nice to share experiences, hear useful tips and learn about various foods that may help build iron. It is nice to get to know and chat with others who are going through some of the same experiences you might be having.

Besides this, make sure you have family and friends around who care for you and love you. Even if they may not be able to relate to what you are experiencing, it is important to have people in your life who care for you to have camaraderie with. Good relationships help to establish a sense of community and will help you feel grounded and balanced. If you lack significant relationships in your life, make sure you reach out to others. As you are feeling better, make it a priority to be around other people. Consider joining a church group, book club, a mom's group or something else. There are many possibilities. The important thing is to find other people you can connect with and have similar interests.

Wholey Cow Affirmations:

I listen to my body and know that persistence pays.
I am taking steps daily to heal my body.

Create Your Own Affirmations:

1. _____
   _____

2. _____
   _____

3. _____
   _____

4. _____
   _____

5. _____
   _____

6. _____
   _____

7. _____
   _____

8. _____
   _____

9. _____
   _____

10. _____
    _____

Glossary of Terms

Clean 15:
A list provided by the Environmental Working Group (EWG) that lists those fruit and vegetables that are considered "clean" and safe to buy conventionally.

Dirty Dozen:
A list provided by the Environmental Working Group (EWG), that lists the top 12 most heavily sprayed produce available.

Dysbiosis:
Dysbiosis is imbalance in the bacteria of the gut, which can cause a variety of health problems and disease.

Enriched Foods:
Enriched foods have nutrients originally found in the product, but were lost during processing added back in to keep some of the original nourishment.

Excitotoxins:
Chemicals (typically amino acids) that over stimulate your brain and can cause neurons to die when there is an overabundance. Some common excitotoxins include MSG (mono-sodium glutamate) and aspartame.

Ferritin:
Ferritin is a blood cell protein. A ferritin test is used to measure the amount of iron your body is storing. If your ferritin level is low, your iron stores are low, indicating you have iron deficiency. The normal ferritin range for men is 20 to 500 nanograms per milliliter (standard units). The normal ferritin range for women is 20 to 200 nanograms per milliliter (standard units).

Fortification:
The process of adding iron or other vitamin and minerals, protein or other ingredient to a product after processing to make it more healthful.

Heme Iron:
Heme iron is found in animals and typically attached to proteins called heme proteins. Heme iron is the best source of iron for people who are iron deficient.

Hemacrit Test:
A hematocrit test measures the percentage of red blood cells in the blood. It is part of a Complete Blood Count (CBC) test and is typically given to diagnosis both anemia and iron deficiency, as well as other vitamin deficiencies, dehydration and some other diseases.

Hydrogenated Oil:
Hydrogenated oil is a man-made oil created using an industrialized process that converts

vegetable oil into a solid form. It is best to limit your intake of these products, as hydrogenated oil has been proven to have ill effects on the body.

Total Iron Binding Capacity (TIBC):
The TIBC test measures the total iron that can be bound to protein in the blood.

Leaky Gut:
Leaky gut happens when the epithelial cells of the intestinal wall break down and cause openings. These openings let food into the bloodstream where they are considered invaders and thus trigger an antibody reaction and inflammation. It also causes malabsorption of nutrients including iron and can lead to other illnesses.

Microbiome:
A microbiome is a community of microorganisms including bacteria, fungi and viruses that inhabit a particular environment, such as in the gut or other area of the human body.

Monosaturated Fats (MUFAS):
MUFAS are the good fats that help your body function optimally. E.g., plant-based foods.

Non Heme Iron:
Non heme iron is found in vegetables, grains and some processed foods. You can also find it in nuts, vegetables, fruit and iron supplements.

Organic Produce:
Organic produce is produce grown without the use of pesticides and harsh chemicals.

Oxalates:
A naturally occurring substance found in vegetables, fruit, nuts and seeds, grain, tea and more. Oxalates help support metabolism, but can cause issues with absorption and may accumulate in the body. It is best to pair them with other foods rich in vitamin C.

Phytates:
Phytates, or phytic acid is a natural combination of elements found in plants. Phytates are typically are found in grains, legumes, nuts and seeds. Although many of these foods are rich in iron, the phytic acid found in them may cause absorption problems. It is best to pair them with foods rich in vitamin C.

Polyphenols:
Polyphenols are chemicals found in plants that give them their coloring. They can be found in wine, chocolate, berries and nuts. It is best to wait an hour or two after having your meal to enjoy a cup of tea or glass of wine.

Serum Iron Test:
A serum iron test measures how much iron is in the serum or liquid of your blood, meaning what is left after both the red blood cells and clotting factors are removed from it.

Tannins:
Tannins are substances that are naturally found in plants, leaves, bark or fruit. They typically have a bitter, acidic taste, yet offer a distinct flavor. Tannins can be found in some tea and wine and may restrict iron absorption in some foods containing iron when consumed together.

Trans-fats:
Trans-fats are found in animals and animal products, such as milk. Other trans-fats are found in a variety of processed foods, such as potato chips, corn chips, crackers, condiments and more.

Transferrin Saturation:
Transferrin saturation shows the percent of transferrin that is saturated with iron.

Transferrin Test:
A transferrin test will measure the direct amount of transferrin found in the blood. Transferrin is a blood cell protein that binds or fastens to iron so it can be transported throughout the body.

Unsaturated Iron Binding Capacity (UIBC):
A UIBC test measures the reserves of transferrin, meaning what has not been saturated with iron.

Serum Ferritin:
A serum ferritin test shows the amount of iron stores in the body.

Recipes

Breakfast

Banana Berry Breakfast Smoothie

1 scoop protein powder (look for one with high iron content)
1 banana
1/2 cup blueberries or blackberries
1 handful spinach or kale
1 tsp. coconut oil
8 oz. cashew or almond milk

Add all ingredients to a Ninja or Vitamix high speed blender, along with a few ice cubes. Blend on high speed until thoroughly blended and mixed. Serve and enjoy. Makes 1 serving.

Black Bean and Sausage Breakfast Burritos

4 large eggs
1/2 cup black beans
1/4 tsp. paprika
1/4 tsp. salt
1/2 lb. spicy Italian sausage
1 cup shredded cheddar cheese
4 (10-in.) flour tortillas
Olive oil

Salsa
1 large avocado cut in small cubes
1/2 cup diced tomatoes
1 small onion, chopped
1 clove garlic, minced
1 Tbsp. fresh lime juice
1/2 tsp. salt
1/4 tsp. ground Cajun
1/4 cup fresh chopped cilantro

In a medium sized bowl, combine the ingredients for the salsa and set aside. In another medium size bowl, whisk the eggs with the smoked paprika and salt. Set aside.

Place the sausage in a large frying pan and cook over medium heat, stirring frequently, until browned (approximately 5 minutes). Drain off any excess grease. Add the black beans and egg mixture to the sausage and continue to cook over low heat, until the eggs are thoroughly cooked. Transfer the sausage and egg mixture to a plate or bowl. Clean the frying pan and place back on the stove. Assemble the burritos by spooning some of the sausage and egg mixture on a tortilla, add approximately 1/4 cup of the salsa mix and top with desired amount of cheese. Next, fold in the sides of the tortilla and roll, tucking in the edges. Lightly coat the frying pan with olive oil and add the burritos, placing seam side down. Cook over medium heat, until the bottoms of the burritos are browned (approximately 3 minutes), then flip. Cook another a few minutes and serve warm.

Chocolate Peanut Butter Delight Smoothie

1 scoop chocolate protein powder (look for one with high iron content)
1 Tbsp. peanut butter
1 tsp. coconut oil
1 handful kale
1 tsp. cacao nibs
8 oz. almond or cashew milk

Add all ingredients to a Ninja or Vitamix high speed blender, along with a few ice cubes. Blend on high speed until thoroughly blended and mixed. Serve and enjoy. Makes 1 serving.

Open Face Breakfast Pizza Sandwich

1 slice sour dough bread
2 Tbsp. pizza sauce
2 breakfast sausage links, cooked to package instructions and cut in slices
6 fresh spinach leaves
Sliced black olives
Garlic powder
Butter
Parmesan cheese

Preheat oven to 350 degrees.

Butter one side of sour dough bread and place it butter side down on a baking sheet. Top with the pizza sauce and spread to cover the edges. Sprinkle with garlic powder over the pizza sauce to taste. Place the spinach leaves on top of the pizza sauce. Add the sausage slices and black olives. Top with parmesan cheese.

Bake in the oven at 350 degrees for 15 minutes or until the cheese is melted and a little crisp.

Pineapple Ginger Juice Blend

1 cup fresh pineapple
1 banana
1 slice fresh ginger
1 handful fresh spinach
2 stalks celery
1 cup water or coconut water

Add all ingredients to a Ninja or Vitamix high speed blender, along with a few ice cubes. Blend on high speed until thoroughly blended and mixed. Serve and enjoy. Makes 1 serving.

Spinach, Tomato & Sausage Frittata

10 large eggs
1/3 cup Parmesan cheese
1/4 cup milk
1/4 tsp. salt
1/4 tsp. pepper
1 package Italian sausage or turkey sausage
4 cups spinach (you can also use kale, or arugula)
Handful cherry tomatoes (sliced in half)
2 Tbsp. fresh chives or 1 small red onion

In a large bowl, lightly whisk together the eggs, cheese, milk, salt and pepper. Set the mixture aside.

In a large frying pan, brown the Italian sausage over medium heat. Stir to break up the meat and cook until slightly crisp. Add the spinach and chives and stir until the spinach is slightly wilted. Remove from heat. Drain off any excess fat from the meat mixture. Set the pan aside.

Spray the bottom of a 9" pie plate with cooking spray. I used an olive oil spray. Pour the meat mixture in the pie plate. Pour the egg mixture over the top of the meat. Top with the cut cherry tomatoes. Place the pie plate in the oven and bake for 25-30 minutes. Let cool for about 5 minutes and then run a paring knife around the inside edges to release the frittata. Cut into wedges and serve warm. You can serve it alone, or with some avocado slices or fresh fruit.

Sides, Salads & Soups

Black Bean, Avocado and Quinoa Rainbow Salad

1 can black beans
1 avocado,cut in cubes
1 large mango, cut in cubes
1/2 tsp. chili, powder
1/2 cup cilantro, chopped
1 clove garlic, minced
1 red bell pepper, chopped
1 small red onion
3/4 cup quinoa
1/2 tsp. salt
1/2 tsp. black pepper
Garlic powder
Turmeric
Olive oil

Dressing
2 Tbsp. olive oil
1 tsp. Dijon mustard
1 Tbsp. honey or maple syrup
2 Tbsp. freshly squeezed lime juice
1 Tbsp. cilantro, chopped
Crushed red pepper

Follow the directions on the package to cook the quinoa. When done, add approximately 1 Tbsp. of olive oil and sprinkle with the salt, pepper, garlic powder and Turmeric. Stir the mix and set aside.

On a large cutting board, chop the vegetables and mango, creating a pile for each one. Place each pile in a section in a large glass bowl, leaving space for the black beans and quinoa. You can add these 2 items first or save them to add last. Set the filled bowl aside.

In a small glass bowl, combine the olive oil, mustard, honey, lime juice, cilantro and crushed red pepper and stir together to make a dressing for the salad. Pour the dressing on top of the rainbow salad and toss together. You can also serve the dressing on the side and serve the salad in the rainbow divided bowl. If you don't like quinoa or eat grains, just skip it and make the salad without it. It is good either way.

Bone Broth

4 quarts water
2 bay leaves
1/4 lb. carrots
1/4 lb. celery
4 cloves garlic
1 medium size onion
1 tsp. pepper
2 tsp. sea salt
2 Tbsp. apple cider vinegar
3 lbs. beef or chicken bones

Place all of the ingredients in a large stockpot or crock pot and bring to a boil. Turn the heat to low and simmer with cover on. Simmer for at least 8 hours. Let cool and strain. Place in containers and store in refrigerator.

Easy Hummus

1/4 cup tahini
1/2 lime (squeeze for juice)
2 Tbsp. olive oil
1 large garlic clove, roughly chopped
Dash paprika
1/2 tsp. salt
1/2 tsp. cumin (optional)
1 (15-ounce) can chickpeas (garbanzo beans) drained and rinsed
2 Tbsp. water
Garnish with chopped fresh herbs (rosemary, parsley, etc.)

Combine the tahini and lime juice in a food processor or high-powered blender, such as a Vitamex. Process the tahini and lime juice for about 2 minutes, pausing to scrape down the bowl of your processor as necessary. Add the chopped garlic, cumin, paprika and salt to the tahini and lime mixture. Blend for about 1 minute. Add the chickpeas to the mix and process for another minute or two. Then add the water and olive oil. Blend the mix for another minute, or until the hummus is thick and smooth. Scrape the hummus into a small serving bowl. Garnish with additional chopped herbs. Serve with fresh vegetables, pita bread or crackers. Store hummus in an airtight container and refrigerate.

Easy Olive Tapenade

1 cup Kalamata olives, pitted and drained
(You can also use half Kalamata olives and half black olives)
2 Tbsp. capers, drained
3-4 Tbsp. olive oil
2 cloves garlic, crushed
1/4 cup fresh parsley, washed and drained well
1 large cucumber, sliced
Parmesan cheese (optional)

Put the olives, capers, garlic and parsley in a blender or food processor and blend until they form a smooth texture. Using a spatula, scrape the mixture into a small bowl and set aside. Place the sliced cucumbers on a plate. Using a teaspoon, spoon some of the Tapenade on each cucumber slice. Garnish with a small spring of parsley.

Note: You can also serve the Tapenade with crackers or some other root vegetable and top with a little Parmesan cheese.

Healthy Strawberry and Cucumber Salad

1 pint strawberries, stemmed and sliced
1 large cucumber, roughly peeled and sliced thin
1/4 cup balsamic vinegar or white balsamic vinegar
1/4 cup honey (you can also use 1/8 tsp. stevia to sweeten, or less. Add to taste.)

In a large bowl, combine the sliced strawberries and cucumbers. Add the balsamic vinegar and honey and stir to coat. Serve immediately or chill for an hour.

Note: You can also add in cilantro or top with slivered almonds.

Double the recipe if you are bringing it to a family gathering or picnic.

Entrees

Chicken Penne with Broccoli and Mushrooms

2 chicken breasts, cut in small pieces
1 small head of broccoli, cut in small florets
1/2 package fresh mushrooms, sliced
1 handful cherry tomatoes, sliced in half
1-2 garlic cloves, crushed
1/2 small onion, chopped
1/2 cup Parmesan cheese
1 (8 oz.) package penne pasta (You can also use pasta made from chick peas.)
Olive oil
Salt
Pepper
Turmeric
Cajun

Fill a large pot with water and bring to boil. Add the penne pasta and reduce heat a little. Cook the pasta for approximately 10 minutes, or until pasta is tender. Remove from heat and strain and then rinse with cool water. Set the pasta aside to cool.

Coat a large skillet with olive oil. Add the chicken pieces and cook over medium heat, until they become slightly crisp. Add the garlic and stir. Add the broccoli, mushrooms and onions and stir. Cover the skillet with a lid and simmer until the vegetables are tender or just a little crisp. Sprinkle with turmeric, salt, pepper and Cajun to taste. Stir the vegetable and chicken mix so it is well coated with the seasoning. Add the sliced cherry tomatoes and Parmesan cheese on the top and stir slightly so tomatoes warm and the cheese starts to melt.

Top with a little more Parmesan cheese, if desired, and serve warm.

Easy Grilled Pesto Chicken

2 pounds boneless skinless chicken breast
Extra-virgin olive oil
1 cup fresh basil, packed (you can most likely find this at a farmers market)
3 cloves garlic
1 cup baby spinach, packed
1/4 cup walnuts
1 cup diced tomatoes
1/2 tsp. salt
Black pepper to taste
Onion powder to taste
1/4 cup grated Parmesan or feta cheese

Toast the garlic and walnuts in a medium-sized pan over medium heat until the outsides of the garlic are lightly browned (approximately 8 minutes). When ready, remove from heat and add garlic and walnuts to a food processor, along with the basil and spinach. Next, add 1/2 teaspoon of salt and process the pesto by pulsing 5 times or so to break down the greens and other ingredients. Then turn the food processor on low speed and slowly drizzle in 1/2 cup olive oil. Blend until the pesto turns to a smooth mix. Add the Parmesan cheese and then process for another 5 seconds or low. Taste and season with additional salt and pepper, if desired. Scrape the mixture in a small glass bowl and set aside.

Drizzle both sides of the chicken breast with olive oil and season with the salt, pepper and onion powder. Place the chicken on a hot grill and flip as each side gets seared and browned. Remove from heat when meat is no longer pink and internal temperature has reached 165°F.

Transfer the chicken breasts to a serving platter. Brush some of the pesto sauce on each chicken breast. Top the chicken with chopped walnuts, tomatoes and cheese. Serve with the extra pesto sauce on the side, along with some fresh asparagus or garden fresh salad.

Easy Asparagus Stuffed Chicken Breasts

2 chicken breasts, sliced down the center
1 bundle of asparagus stalks, cut in half
Garlic powder
Paprika
Turmeric
Salt and pepper
Avocado oil
Parmesan cheese (Add to taste)

Slice the chicken breasts, so they are almost sliced in half (butterflied). Coat the bottom of a large frying pan with avocado oil. Place the sliced chicken breasts in the pan and brown on medium heat. Season with salt, pepper, garlic powder, turmeric and paprika, and flip. When they are evenly browned, remove the pan from the heat and set aside. Using a fork, remove the chicken and place on a foil-lined baking sheet. You can also use a glass baking pan. Sprinkle the chicken with the crushed garlic. Add a handful of the asparagus (I used 4-5 spears per chicken breast). Top with some Parmesan cheese to taste. Fold the other side of chicken over. Use a couple of tooth picks to hold the chicken together. Do the same for the other chicken breast. Bake at 350 degrees for 25 to 30 minutes or until internal temperature of chicken has reached 165°F.

Easy Cashew Chicken Stir Fry

1 Tbsp. avocado oil
1 lb. boneless skinless chicken breasts, cut into 1-inch pieces
Salt and pepper, to taste
3 cloves garlic, minced
2 cups broccoli florets
1 red bell pepper, sliced
1 green bell pepper, sliced
3/4 cup zucchini, sliced
1/2 cup carrots, chopped
1/3 cup unsalted cashews

Sauce

4 Tbsp. tamari (or soy sauce)
3 Tbsp. all-natural peanut butter
2 Tbsp. honey
1 tsp. sesame oil
1 Tbsp. grated ginger
2 or 3 Tbsp. water

In a small bowl, whisk together tamari (or soy sauce), peanut butter, honey, sesame oil and grated ginger to make the sauce. Add 2 or 3 tablespoons of water to the mix to make desired consistency you prefer, and set aside.

In a large skillet, drizzle avocado oil and add chicken. Season with salt and pepper and sauté until the chicken is browned. Add the garlic and sauté for approximately 30 seconds or so, mixing it with the chicken.

Add broccoli, bell pepper, red pepper, onion, zucchini slices and carrots to the skillet with the chicken and mix everything together. Cook an additional 5 minutes, or until the veggies are tender. Top with the cashews and serve alone or with rice.

Easy Garlic Honey and Lime Shrimp

1 lb. shelled and de-veined shrimp
1 Tbsp. olive oil
1 Tbsp. melted butter
4 cloves garlic, minced
3 Tbsp. honey
1 & 1/2 Tbsp. fresh lime juice
1/4 tsp. salt
Cayenne pepper
Fresh thyme, chopped
Fresh dill, chopped
Fresh parsley, chopped

Rinse the shrimp with cold water, drain and then set aside.

In a large skillet, add the olive oil and melt the butter over medium heat. Add the garlic and sauté until it turns slightly brown. Add the shrimp and stir a few times. Add the honey, lime juice, salt and cayenne pepper to the mix, as well as the chopped dill and thyme. Cook the shrimp until the honey lime mix thickens up. Remove from heat. Serve with vegetables and rice, if desired. Garnish the shrimp with the chopped parsley.

Easy Spinach Parmesan Squash Noodles

Butternut squash spirals (10.7 oz. package or make your own)
2 Tbsp. butter
2 cloves garlic, minced
2 cups packed spinach
1/4 cup freshly grated Parmesan cheese
Salt and black pepper, to taste

In a large skillet, melt the butter over medium-high heat. Add the garlic and cook for 1-2 minutes or until slightly brown. Add in the butternut squash noodles and spinach. Gently toss and cook until spinach leaves are wilted, about 2-3 minutes. Stir in 1/4 cup of the Parmesan cheese and toss until butternut squash noodles are coated in the Parmesan cheese. Add salt and the ground black pepper to taste. Remove from heat and serve warm.

Easy Sausage Spinach Vegetable Lasagna

1 small box lasagna noodles (1/2 lb. or approximately 9 noodles)
(Note: You can use a gluten-free variety if you have issues with gluten.)
1 (24 oz.) jar spaghetti sauce
1 container (22 oz.) cottage cheese or ricotta cheese
2-3 cups shredded mozzarella or cheddar cheese
1 lb. Italian sausage (omit if you prefer a meatless version of lasagna)
1/2 bag of fresh spinach or kale
1 small red onion, diced
1 small green pepper, chopped
1 small package fresh mushrooms
1 small can black olives
1/2 jar green olives
1-2 cloves garlic, minced
2 medium size tomatoes, diced
Salt and pepper
Cajun seasoning

Pre-heat oven to 350 degrees.

Boil a large pot of water and add the lasagna noodles. Turn down heat a bit and boil the noodles for 10 minutes, strain off the water and set aside.

In a large skillet, brown the Italian sausage. Add the garlic, onion, green pepper and mushrooms. Stir the mixture until the vegetables are slightly browned. Add in the olives and the salt, pepper and Cajun seasoning to taste and stir. Add the spaghetti sauce to the meat and vegetable mix and stir to combine all of the ingredients. Add the tomatoes to the top and stir, just so they become warm, and then remove from the heat.

Grease a 13" x 9" cake pan with olive oil. Place 3 noodles on the bottom of the pan. Then spoon about 1/3 of the meat and vegetable sauce over the noodles. Grab a handful or so of the spinach and place it on top of the sauce. Next scoop about 1/3 of the cottage cheese on top of the spinach and then add a layer of the mozzarella or cheddar cheese. Repeat these steps 2 more times to create 3 layers total. Place the prepared pan of lasagna in the oven and bake for 30-40, or until slightly crisp on the top. Remove from the oven and let set and cool for another 30-45 minutes. Serve warm with a fresh garden salad.

Fried Sauerkraut

2-4 Tbsp. butter, ghee or olive oil
2 cups sauerkraut, drained
2 slices cooked bacon or turkey bacon, cut in small pieces
Salt and pepper to taste

In a large frying pan, add the butter or other oil and melt or warm. Add the sauerkraut and sauté until lightly browned. Add the bacon pieces. Season the mix with the salt and pepper to taste. Serve warm alone or as a side dish.

Note: You can also add a handful of fresh spinach to the mix while sautéing the sauerkraut.

Grilled Satay Chicken with Peanut Sauce

2 lbs. chicken breasts, sliced into 1/2-1" strips*
2 Tbsp. olive oil
1/4 cup smooth peanut butter
20-30 wooden skewers

Marinade Sauce

1/4 cup low sodium soy sauce
1/4 cup packed brown sugar or Coconut Palm sugar
1 Tbsp. chili paste
1 & 1/2 Tbsp. lime juice
1 & 1/2 Tbsp. Hoisin sauce
1 tsp. dried basil
1 tsp. cumin powder
1/2 tsp. ground ginger
1/2 tsp. garlic powder
1/2 tsp. turmeric powder

In a medium bowl, whisk together the Marinade Sauce ingredients. Measure a 1/4 cup of the mix and pour into a freezer size bag along with 2 tablespoons olive oil. Add the chicken and toss to evenly coat. Store the chicken and marinade mix in the refrigerator 6 hours or overnight. Refrigerate the remaining marinade/sauce separately, as this will become the base of your Peanut Sauce.

When ready to cook, soak wooden skewers in water for at least 30 minutes.

Meanwhile, remove chicken from refrigerator to bring to room temperature. Thread chicken onto skewers and lightly dab excess marinade off with paper towels.

Grease an indoor or outdoor grill and heat to medium heat. Once the grill is hot, place the skewers of chicken on grill and leave on for approximately 4 minutes per side, or until chicken is cooked through.

Add reserved marinade sauce to a small saucepan and bring it to a boil. Simmer for 1 minute. Remove from heat then stir in 1/4 cup peanut butter until completely combined. If the sauce is too thick, you can stir in water 1 tablespoon at a time, until it is the desired consistency. Taste and add additional chili sauce or peanut butter, if desired.

Serve chicken warm with Peanut Sauce for an appetizer or serve with rice and veggies for a main course.

Healthy Chicken Parmesan Kale Pasta

2 medium size chicken breasts, grilled and sliced
1 bunch (about 1/2 lb.) kale
1/2 lb. angel hair pasta (you can also use a gluten free option)
2 Tbsp. olive oil
2 Tbsp. butter
2 cloves garlic, minced
1/2 package mushrooms, sliced (about 4 oz.)
1/4 cup grated Parmesan
Cherry tomatoes (handful or 2 sliced in half)
Salt & pepper
Red pepper flakes

Season the chicken with salt and pepper and other favorite seasoning. Place the chicken on a heated grill and cook until done, flipping the meat as needed. When the chicken is done, remove from heat and let cool slightly. Slice the chicken in thin strips and set aside.

Bring a large pot of water to a boil. Break the pasta in half, add it to the boiling water and cook until soft (about 10 minutes). Drain the pasta in a colander. While the pasta is cooking, add the olive oil, butter, minced garlic and sliced mushrooms in a large skillet pan. Cook over medium heat for 1-2 minutes, or until the garlic is soft and mushrooms slightly browned. Add the washed kale and continue to sauté until the kale has slightly wilted. Add the sliced chicken. Add the drained pasta to the kale mix. Toss the pasta and kale together. Season the pasta and kale with salt and pepper to taste and then add the red pepper flakes. Add the sliced cherry tomatoes and stir to warm. Top with the grated Parmesan cheese.

Healthy Sesame Chicken

1 lb. boneless skinless chicken breasts, cut into 1/2 inch strips
2 Tbsp. cornstarch
1 pinch salt & pepper or to taste
Garlic powder to taste
1 Tbsp. olive oil
Small bunch onion scallions, chopped
Cooked rice for serving (I like to use Jasmine or Basmati rice)

Sauce
3 Tbsp. soy sauce
2 Tbsp. honey
1 tsp. sriracha or to taste
1 tsp. fresh ginger, grated
1 clove garlic, minced
2 Tbsp. sesame seeds
1 Tbsp. sesame oil

In a medium bowl, combine the soy sauce, honey, sriracha, ginger, garlic, sesame seeds and sesame oil. Set aside.

In a large bowl combine the chicken, cornstarch, salt, pepper and garlic. In a large frying pan, add the olive oil and heat for approximately 2 minutes on medium heat. Add the chicken and stir-fry for about 5 minutes or until the chicken is golden brown and cooked through. Add the prepared sauce and allow it to simmer for 3-4 minutes, or until the sauce is thick and slightly sticky.

Remove the chicken from the pan and sprinkle with chopped onions, if desired. Sprinkle with more sesame seeds to garnish. Serve alone or with your favorite rice and side salad.

Healthy Thai Chicken Salad

1 Tbsp. Coconut oil
1 small red onion chopped fine
2 cloves garlic, minced
1 lb. boneless skinless chicken breasts, chopped into small chunks
2 Tbsp. lime juice (1/2 fresh lime juiced)
3 Tbsp. Tamari soy sauce
1 Tbsp. fresh ginger peeled and grated
2 tsp. red pepper flakes
1 Tbsp. honey
3 Tbsp. extra virgin olive oil
4 cups shredded cabbage (red or green)
1 red pepper diced
3 carrots grated
1/4 cup fresh parsley chopped
1/4 cup fresh cilantro chopped
1/4-1/2 cup chopped spinach
1/4 cup cashews

In a large frying pan, heat the coconut oil over medium heat. Season the chicken to taste with the salt and pepper. Add the onion and garlic and cook for approximately two minutes. Add the chicken and sauté until it is browned and fully cooked. Remove from heat and set it aside.

Dressing

In a small bowl, whisk together the lime juice, Tamari soy sauce, ginger and red pepper flakes. Slowly whisk in the olive oil and blend until olive oil is mixed in with the other ingredients. Add the honey to taste.

Salad

In a large bowl, combine the cabbage, red pepper, carrots, parsley, spinach, cilantro and chicken. Toss with the dressing or serve dressing on the side. Top with cashews.

Home Made Tacos

1 lb. hamburger or ground turkey
1 small can (2.25 oz.) black olives, sliced
1 small red onion, chopped

In a frying pan, brown the hamburger or turkey over medium high heat. Add the onion and cook until browned. Add the sliced olives. When the hamburger is completely browned, add in 2 tablespoons of the prepared taco seasoning below, along with 3/4 cup water. Stir the mix until well combined and then remove from heat.

Home-Made Taco Seasoning Mix

1/2 tsp. garlic powder, organic
1/2 tsp. onion powder, organic
1/2 tsp. oregano, organic
2 Tbsp. chili powder, organic
1 tsp. paprika, organic
2 tsp. pepper, organic
1/2 tsp. red pepper flakes, organic
2 & 1/2 tsp. salt
1 Tbsp. cumin, organic

In a small bowl, measure all of the spices. Store them in a glass jar in your cupboard to have on hand the next time you want to make tacos. Feel free to substitute other spices you like.

Use 2 tablespoons of the mix per 1 pound of hamburger, turkey or chicken. Add 3/4 cup of water to blend the spices in with the meat.

Mediterranean Seared Salmon

4 small salmon fillets or 2 large fillets
Olive oil
1 tsp. paprika
1 tsp. garlic powder
1/2 tsp. onion powder
1/2 tsp. ground cumin
1/4 tsp. salt
1/4 tsp black pepper
Pinch cayenne pepper
Cajun seasoning to taste
1 tsp. fresh lime juice

Place the salmon fillets in a large bowl or large Ziploc bag. Add 2 tablespoons of olive oil. Next add the paprika, garlic powder, onion powder, cumin, salt, pepper, cayenne, Cajun seasoning and lime juice. Toss until the fillets are well-coated and then let the salmon marinate for at least 20 minutes or longer. For more flavor, you can marinate the fillets overnight.

When the salmon is marinated, coat a large cast-iron skillet with 2-3 tablespoons of olive oil. When the oil is hot, add the salmon fillets and sear for about 4 minutes, or until they are a golden-brown. Using a large metal spatula, flip the fillets and allow them to cook and sear on the other side for another 4 more minutes and remove them from skillet.

Mediterranean Salsa

1 cup small cherry or sugar tomatoes, quartered
1 small cucumber, diced
1/4 yellow bell pepper, diced
2 Tbsp. pitted Kalamata or black olives, diced
2 Tbsp. red onion, diced
1 tsp. parsley, chopped
1/2 tsp. lime juice
Salt to taste
Black pepper to taste

In a small bowl, combine all of the ingredients. Use a spoon to mix and combine the ingredients. Top the salmon fillets with the salsa mix. Serve alone or with rice, quinoa or vegetable.

Rosemary and Sea Salt Sweet Potato Fries

1 Tbsp. Rosemary, fresh cut
1 sweet potato, large
1/2 tsp. paprika, smoked
1 tsp. sea salt
3 Tbsp. olive oil

Pre-heat the oven to 350 degrees.

Cut the sweet potato into long French fry-shaped pieces and place them in a large mixing bowl. Add the paprika, sea salt, rosemary and olive oil. Feel free to add any other spices you like such as pepper or garlic. Using a large spoon, mix all the ingredients together until the potatoes are well coated.

Spread the fries evenly on a large baking sheet and place in the oven. Bake for 20 minutes and then flip to crisp up the other side. Bake for an additional 20 minutes or until the fries are golden. Remove from the oven and serve immediately.

Spiral Meatloaf

1/4 cup onion, diced
1/4 cup green pepper, diced
1 can (2.25 oz.) black olives
1/2 tsp. garlic
1 tsp. oil
1/3 cup spaghetti sauce or BBQ sauce
1/3 cup bread crumbs
1 egg
1/2-3/4 tsp. garlic salt
1 lb. lean ground beef
3/4 cup shredded cheddar cheese or other variety
2 Tbsp. Parmesan cheese

Pre-heat oven to 350 degrees.

Sauté onion, pepper, garlic and black olives in oil over medium heat. Set aside. In a bowl, combine the bread crumbs, egg, 2 tablespoons spaghetti sauce and salt, and blend together. Add the beef and mix with your hands. On waxed paper, shape the meat into a 12" x 8" rectangle. Sprinkle the cooked vegetables over the meat.

Bake for 1 hour. Spread the remaining sauce over the top and bake another 10 minutes.

Note: Feel free to add in other vegetables including a handful or two of spinach or kale, jalapeno peppers, mushrooms, etc.

Warm Spinach and Feta Salad with Black Beans

2 large handfuls fresh spinach (approximately 1/2 prepared bag)
1 small red onion, chopped
1/2 can (15 oz.) black beans
6-8 cherry tomatoes, halved
1 clove garlic, crushed
1 handful feta cheese crumbles (add to taste)
Avocado, cut in slices
Cajun seasoning
Turmeric
Soy sauce or coconut aminos

Coat the bottom of a large frying pan with olive oil. Add the spinach, onion, and garlic. Stir on medium heat, until the onion begins to brown and the spinach is slightly wilted. Sprinkle with turmeric and Cajun seasoning. Add the tomatoes and stir slightly, until they are just warm. Spoon the salad on a plate. Add the feta cheese on top. Serve with avocado slices and any other garnish you may like. Top with a little coconut aminos or soy sauce, if desired.

Desserts

Chocolate Coconut Energy Balls

3/4 cup cashews
2 Tbsp. cocoa powder
1/2 Tbsp. coconut oil
12 pitted Medjool dates
3/4 cup coconut milk
2 Tbsp. coconut Flakes
1/2 tsp. salt

Place the cashews in a food processor or high speed blender, such as a Vitamix, to crush. Pulse until the nuts are evenly crushed. Next add your cocoa powder, coconut oil, dates, coconut milk and coconut flakes and blend well, until the mixture forms a thick paste.

Use a spoon to scoop out enough of the mixture to form a round ball. You can roll the balls in coconut flakes or dip them in cocoa powder. Place the prepared balls in a cake pan lined with parchment paper, or place on a cutting board. Place the pan in the freezer for an hour or more to firm and serve. Store the balls in air-tight container in the freezer.

Chocolate Coconut Peanut Butter Energy Balls

1 cup chopped nuts (pecans, walnuts, hazelnuts, etc.)
2/3 cup coconut flakes (I used an organic version)
1/2 cup peanut butter (I used a natural brand with less sugar)
1/2 cup ground flaxseed
3/4 cup dark chocolate chips (you can also use mini-chocolate chips)
1/3 cup raw honey
1 tsp. vanilla extract

In a medium size bowl, combine all of the ingredients and mix together, until thoroughly combined. Place the dough in the refrigerator for about a half an hour. Shape into 1-inch balls. Store the balls in an air-tight container in the refrigerator.

Chocolate Date and Nut Energy Bites

1/2 cup ground raw pumpkin seeds (you can also use sunflower or sesame seeds)

1/2 cup ground flax seeds

1/2 cup raw cashew nuts (you can also use Brazil nuts or almonds)

1 & 1/2 cups of Medjool dates (make sure the pits are removed)

4 oz. dark chocolate (I used a brand with a high cacao content. Look for 62% to 72% cacao content for the most nutritional benefit)

1 Tbsp. coconut oil

Place the first 4 ingredients into a food processor and blend until they stick to the side of the bowl. Next, roll the mix into evenly formed balls and place them on a cookie sheet lined with parchment paper. Set aside.

Melt the chocolate chips and coconut oil in a double boiler. If you don't have a double boiler, you can also use 2 different size pots. Fill the larger pot with water and bring to a boil. Add the chocolate chips and coconut oil in the smaller pot and place on the surface of the boiling water. Stir the chocolate and coconut oil, until it is melted. Remove from heat and let it cool slightly. Using a spoon, dip the balls in the chocolate to cover completely. Place them back on the parchment paper to set. Place the cookie sheet in the refrigerator for at least 30 minutes or until the chocolate is hardened.

Chocolate Zucchini Bread

2, 1 oz. chocolate squares
3 eggs
1 cup sugar (you can also use coconut palm sugar for a lower glycemic load)
1/2 cup honey (you can substitute 1 cup of honey and omit the sugar)
1 cup oil (I used olive oil)
2 cups grated zucchini
3 cups flour (you can substitute rice flour if you are looking for a gluten free option)
1 tsp. soda
1 tsp. salt
1 tsp. cinnamon
1 bag dark chocolate chips

Preheat oven to 350 degrees.

Lightly grease two loaf pans. Using a double boiler, melt the chocolate squares. If you don't have a double boiler, you can also use 2 different size pots. Fill the larger pot with water and bring to a boil. Add the chocolate and place on the surface of the boiling water.Stir until smooth and set aside. In a large mixing bowl, mix the eggs, sugar, honey, oil, zucchini and vanilla. Add the melted chocolate and mix until smooth. Add the baking soda, salt and cinnamon. Fold in the flour. Add the chocolate chips. Pour the batter in the two loaf pans. Bake at 350 degrees for approximately 60 minutes, or until a toothpick poked in the center comes out clean.

Easy Chocolate Avocado Truffles

1 avocado, mashed
3/4 cup dark chocolate chips (the higher cacao content the better)
1/2 tsp. vanilla extract
Pinch of cinnamon
1-2 tsp. of cocoa powder to coat

Melt the chocolate using a double boiler. You can also use 2 different sized pots. Fill the one with water and bring it to a boil on the stove. Put the smaller pot on top of the boiling water and add the chocolate. Stir the chocolate, until it is completely melted and has a smooth consistency. Set aside.

In a another bowl, mash the avocado. Add the melted chocolate and stir until they are combined and free of clumps. Next add in the vanilla and cinnamon. Place the mixture in the refrigerator for about 30 minutes or so. When the mix is cooled and slightly firm, use a spoon to scoop and roll into balls. Roll the prepared balls in cocoa powder and serve.

Note: You can also roll them in coconut flakes.

If you have any left-over truffles, you can store them in an air tight container in the refrigerator.

Easy Pumpkin Muffins

1 & 3/4 cups all-purpose flour (you can also use almond flour or rice flour if you want to avoid gluten)
1 cup sugar (you can substitute 1 tsp. powder or liquid stevia for the sugar if you want)
1/2 cup dark brown sugar (I used coconut palm sugar)
1 tsp. baking soda
1/2 tsp. salt
2 tsp. cinnamon
1/4 tsp. ginger
1/4 tsp. nutmeg
2 eggs
1 (15 oz.) can pure pumpkin
1/2 cup coconut oil
1 tsp. vanilla extract

Preheat the oven to 350 degrees.

Place 12 paper liners into standard size muffin baking pan cups. Measure the flour, sugar, baking soda, salt and spices into a medium bowl and mix together. Set the bowl aside. In a mixer, add the eggs, pumpkin, coconut oil and vanilla extract. Mix at a medium speed until well blended. Add the dry ingredients to the mixture. Mix until all of the dry ingredients are blended in the batter. Using a large spoon, scoop the batter into the paper liners. Bake for 20 minutes or until a toothpick inserted into the center of a muffin comes out clean. Serve warm or let them cool and serve later.

Molasses Muffins

1 cup flour
1/2 cup ground flax seed
1 tsp. baking powder
1 tsp. baking soda
1/4 tsp. salt
1 & 1/2 tsp. cinnamon
1 tsp. ginger
1/2 tsp. nutmeg
2 eggs
2/3 cup unsulphured molasses
1 apple, peeled and grated
1 carrot, grated
1/2 cup walnuts, chopped
1 cup golden raisins
1/4 cup coconut oil

Preheat oven to 350 degrees.

Line a muffin pan with 12 paper liners.

Combine the flour, flax seed, baking soda, baking powder, salt, cinnamon, ginger, and nutmeg in a large bowl and set aside.

In a mixing bowl, mix the eggs, molasses, apple, carrot, walnuts and coconut oil together on low speed. Add the flour mixture and mix thoroughly, until all combined. Spoon the mix into the muffin tins and bake for about 18 minutes, or until a toothpick inserted in the middle of a muffin comes out clean.

Note: This recipe has no added sugar. It gets its light sweetness from the molasses, apples, carrots and raisins. If you prefer a little more sweetness, you can add 1/2 cup of sugar or coconut palm sugar.

About The Author

Barbara Rodgers is the author of *Wholey Cow A Simple Guide To Eating And Living*, and is a Certified Integrative Health Coach. She is a former small business owner and has a B.S. in Mass Communications.

After developing iron deficiency, Barbara wanted to learn more about nutrition to help re-gain her health and enrolled at the Institute for Integrative Nutrition® where she learned over a hundred different dietary theories. Using this knowledge, she enjoys spreading the word about eating the right food, exercising and creating balance to live a healthy lifestyle. She is passionate about helping people get healthy and stay healthy.

Barbara loves to cook and bake and enjoys sharing meals with family and friends. She finds joy spending time with her husband, family and grand-children. She also enjoys time spent at the lake and likes to read, write and exercise.

Connect With Barbara!

barbararodgersonline.com
Instagram: @barb.rodgers
Facebook: Barbara Rodgers Health Coach

Resources

[1]"Iron Deficiency Anemia Secondary to Inadequate Dietary Iron Intake." Healthline, Healthline Media, www.healthline.com/health/iron-deficiency-inadequate-dietary-iron.

[2]"Panic Attacks and Anxiety Episodes Linked to Vitamin Deficiencies in Groundbreaking Study." Awareness Act, 26 Jan. 2019, awarenessact.com/panic-attackss-and-anxiety-episodes-linked-to-vitamin-deficiencies-in-groundbreaking-study/.

[3]Zwillich, Todd. "Mild Iron Deficiency May Harm Women's Memory." WebMD, WebMD, www.webmd.com/women/news/20040419/mild-iron-deficiency-may-harm-womens-memory.

[4] "Heavy Metal: Iron and the Brain." Psychology Today, Sussex Publishers, www.psychologytoday.com/us/blog/evolutionary-psychiatry/201511/heavy-metal-iron-and-the-brain.

[5]"22 Shocking Iron Deficiency Anemia Statistics." HRF, 3 Aug. 2018, healthresearchfunding.org/22-shocking-iron-deficiency-anemia-statistics/.

[6]"What Is Iron?" Idi, www.irondisorders.org/what-is-iron.

[7]"The Role of Iron in the Body." Spatone, 1 Jan. 1AD, www.spatone.com/info-hub/the-role-of-iron-in-the-body.

[8]"Do You Know What Is the Role of Iron in the Human Body?" YouTube, YouTube, 11 Apr. 2017, www.youtube.com/watch?v=XVIKtzCS6jk&t=23s.

[9]FAAEM, Darin Ingels ND. "Iron Deficiency: More Common Than You Might Think." Dr. Darin Ingels, ND FAAEM, Dr. Darin Ingels, ND FAAEM, 24 Jan. 2019, dariningelsnd.com/iron-deficiency-more-common-than-you-might-think/.

[10] "Ferritin Test." Mayo Clinic, Mayo Foundation for Medical Education and Research, 10 Feb. 2017, www.mayoclinic.org/Tests-Procedures/Ferritin-Test/about/Pac-20384928.

[11]"Fatigue? Anxiety? Insomnia? Could Be Iron Deficiency." Amber Wood Health, 3 Dec. 2018, amberwoodhealth.ca/fatigue-anxiety-insomnia-could-be-iron-deficiency/.

[12]Dionisio, Kara, and David Miller. "That Naturopathic Podcast: Ironman. The World's Most Common Nutrient Deficiency Is Still a Problem on Apple Podcasts." Apple Podcasts, 19 Apr. 2019, podcasts.apple.com/us/podcast/ironman-worlds-most-common-nutrient-deficiency-is-still/id1450694474?i=1000435518141.

[13]Soppi, Esa T. "Iron Deficiency without Anemia - a Clinical Challenge." Clinical Case Reports, John Wiley and Sons Inc., 17 Apr. 2018, www.ncbi.nlm.nih.gov/pmc/articles/PMC5986027/

[14]"Hematocrit Test." Mayo Clinic, Mayo Foundation for Medical Education and Research, 12 Feb. 2019, www.mayoclinic.org/tests-procedures/hematocrit/about/pac-20384728.

[15] "Iron Tests." Patient Education on Blood, Urine, and Other Lab Tests, labtestsonline.org/tests/iron-tests.

[16] "Iron Deficiency Anemia." Mayo Clinic, Mayo Foundation for Medical Education and Research, 11 Nov. 2016, www.mayoclinic.org/diseases-conditions/iron-deficiency-anemia/symptoms-causes/syc-20355034.

[17]"Can Iron Every (Other) Day Keep the Doctor Away?", 2 Feb. 2018, www.hematology.org/Thehematologist/Diffusion/8265.aspx.

[18]"Why Managing Your Iron Level Is Crucial to Your Health." Mercola.com, articles.mercola.com/sites/articles/archive/2017/05/31/managing-iron-levels.aspx.

[19]Childs, Westin. "7 Reasons to Treat Low Ferritin Levels + Step-by-Step Treatment Guide." Dr. Westin Childs | Thyroid & Health Supplements That Work, 12 Feb. 2019, www.restartmed.com/low-ferritin/.

[20]Dionisio, Kara, and David Miller. "That Naturopathic Podcast: Ironman. The World's Most Common Nutrient Deficiency Is Still a Problem on Apple Podcasts." Apple Podcasts, 19 Apr. 2019, podcasts.apple.com/us/podcast/ironman-worlds-most-common-nutrient-deficiency-is-still/id1450694474?i=1000435518141.

[21]Johnson, Brian. "Grass Fed Beef SPLEEN - $44." Grass Fed Desiccated Spleen, ancestralsupplements.com/spleen.

[22]"Do You Absorb More Iron Cooking in a Cast Iron Pan?" Runners Connect, 9 May 2016, runnersconnect.net/cast-iron-pan-iron/.

[23] "Food Fortification." Wikipedia, Wikimedia Foundation, 5 Aug. 2019, en.wikipedia.org/wiki/Food_fortification.

[24]Ferreira, Mandy. "Are fortified and Enriched Foods Healthy." Healthline. https://www.healthline.com/health/food-nutrition/fortified-and-enriched-foods#2.

[25]"Fortified Food Fraud." Feeding You Lies: How to Unravel the Food Industry's Playbook and Reclaim Your Health, by Vani Hari, Hay House, Inc., 2019, pp. 158–158.

[26]"Iron We Consume." Idi, www.irondisorders.org/Iron-We-Consume.

[27]"Top Iron-Rich Foods List." WebMD, WebMD, www.webmd.com/diet/iron-rich-foods.

[28]"Shopper's Guide To Pesticides In Produce." www.ewg.org/foodnews/August, 2019.

[29] "Home - PubMed - NCBI." National Center for Biotechnology Information, U.S. National Library of Medicine, www.ncbi.nlm.nih.gov/pubmed.

[30]"Good Fats vs. Bad Fats: Dr. Hyman's Healthy Cheat Sheet." The Chalkboard, 11 Mar. 2016, thechalkboardmag.com/dr-hyman-good-fat-bad-fat.

[31]"EXCITOTOXINS – By Dr. Russell L. Blaylock, MD." EXCITOTOXINS, www.joyfulaging.com/Excitotoxins.htm.

[32]"Over 34 Hidden Names for MSG." Foods That Heal You, 9 Jan. 2019, foodsthathealyou.com/over-34-hidden-names-for-msg/.

[33]Wei, Emily. "The Myth of the Nutrition Facts Label – Iron Absorption Debunked." The Myth of the Nutrition Facts Label – Iron Absorption Debunked, blog.insidetracker.com/blood-levels-vs.-food-labels-what-everybody-ought-to-know-about-iron.

[34]Nandy, Priyadarshini. "8 Amazing Apricot Benefits: The Nutritional Heavyweight Among Fruits." Food.ndtv.com. N.p., 19 Apr. 2016. Web. 16 May 2017.

[35]"How to Tend to Your Inner Garden – Why Your Gut Flora May Be Making You Sick." Dr. Mark Hyman, 8 Jan. 2015, drhyman.com/blog/2014/10/10/tend-inner-garden-gut-flora-may-making-sick/.

[36]Sonnenburg, Justin Sonnenburg Erica. "Gut Feelings–the 'Second Brain' in Our Gastrointestinal Systems [Excerpt]." Scientific American, 1 May 2015, www.scientificamerican.com/article/gut-feelings-the-second-brain-in-our-gastrointestinal-systems-excerpt/.

[37]"Microbiome." Merriam-Webster, Merriam-Webster, www.merriam webster.com/dictionary/microbiome.

[38]"What's the Gut Got To Do With It?" Women's Voice, 26 Apr. 2018, womensvoicemagazine.com/whats-the-gut-got-to-do-with-it.

[39]"Anemia–The Real Cause & Why More Iron Will Make the Problem Worse." Healthy Families for God, 21 May 2017, www.healthyfamiliesforgod.com/blog/2017/05/anemia-the-real-iron-problem-worse.

[40]Harvard Health Publishing. "Ask Dr. Rob about Vitamin B12 Deficiency." Harvard Health, www.health.harvard.edu/staying-healthy/ask-dr-rob-about-vitamin-b12-deficiency.

[41]Ruggeri, Christine. "Vitamin B12 Benefits That You're Probably Missing." Dr. Axe, 28 Sept. 2018, draxe.com/vitamin-b12-benefits/.

[42]"Vitamin Deficiency Anemia." Mayo Clinic, Mayo Foundation for Medical Education and Research, 9 Nov. 2016, www.mayoclinic.org/diseases-conditions/vitamin-deficiency-anemia/symptoms-causes/syc-20355025.

[43]Myers, Amy. "Everything You Need To Know About B12 Deficiency." Amy Myers MD, 31 July 2018, www.amymyersmd.com/2013/08/everything-need-know-b12-deficiency/.

[44]Myers, Amy. "This Is Your Gut On Gluten." Amy Myers MD, 27 July 2018, www.amymyersmd.com/2016/05/your-gut-on-gluten/.

[45]Neslen, Arthur. "Glyphosate Shown to Disrupt Microbiome 'at Safe Levels', Study Claims." The Guardian, Guardian News and Media, 16 May 2018, www.theguardian.com/environment/2018/may/16/glyphosate-shown-to-disrupt-microbiome-at-safe-levels-study-claims.

[46]"New Studies Reveal Damaging Effects of Glyphosate." Mercola.com, 15 April 2014. articles.mercola.com/sites/articles/archive/2014/04/15/glyphosate-health-effects.aspx.

[47]"Glyphosate Binds Vital Nutrients." The Detox Project, detoxproject.org/glyphosate/glyphosate-chelating-agent/.

[48]Suzuki, Wendy. "The Brain-Changing Benefits of Exercise." TED, www.ted.com/talks/wendy_suzuki_the_brain_changing_benefits_of_exercise?language=en.

[49]Wells, Katie. "How to Use Red Raspberry Leaf Herb: Wellness Mama." Wellness Mama®, wellnessmama.com/5107/raspberry-leaf/.

[50]"Essential Oils for Anemia- Boost Red Blood Cell Production." The Nutri Guide, 15 May 2019, thenutriguide.com/essential-oils-for-anemia/.

[51]Wells, Katie. "Frankincense Oil Uses and Benefits: Wellness Mama." Wellness Mama®, wellnessmama.com/123712/frankincense-oil-uses-benefits/.

[52]Lade, Heiko, and Heiko LadeBased. "Acupuncture for Anemia." The Acupuncture Clinic, 29 Mar. 2019, www.theacupunctureclinic.co.nz/acupuncture-for-anemia/.

[53]Sissons, Claire. "L-Theanine: Benefits, Risks, Sources, and Dosage." Medical News Today, MediLexicon International, www.medicalnewstoday.com/articles/324120.php.

[54]"Using Affirmations: – Harnessing Positive Thinking." Stress Management From MindTools.com, www.mindtools.com/pages/article/affirmations.htm.

[55]"Benjamin Franklin Quote." A, www.azquotes.com/quote/101922.

[56] "Francis Bacon Quote." A, www.azquotes.com/quote/14782.

[57]Daily Inspirational Quotes. "Strength Doesn't Come from What You Can Do. It Comes from..." Daily Inspirational Quotes, 27 July 2016, www.dailyinspirationalquotes.in/2016/07/strength-doesnt-come-can-comes-overcoming-things-thought-couldnt-rikki-rogers/.

[58]Projects, Contributors to Wikimedia. "Cartoon Fictional Character." Wikiquote, Wikimedia Foundation, Inc., 30 May 2019, en.wikiquote.org/wiki/Popeye.

[59] "Hippocrates Quote." A, www.azquotes.com/quote/823835.

[60]"Kenneth H. Cooper Quote." A, www.azquotes.com/quote/785940.

[61]"Pablo Picasso Quote." A, www.azquotes.com/quote/231314.

Also by Barbara Rodgers

The Amazon bestseller, *Wholey Cow A Simple Guide To Eating And Living*, is a useful guide for anyone looking to live a healthy life style. Learn 7 Guiding Principles to Help You Eat Well and Live Well!

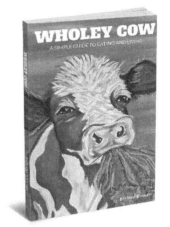

1. Food is Fuel
2. Know Thyself
3. Reach for Rainbow Colors
4. Less is More!
5. Quality vs. Quantity—Make Conscious Choices
6. Ask What's Missing
7. Take Charge

Made in the USA
Monee, IL
08 September 2021

77681699R00081